# BACKYARD
# MEDICINE

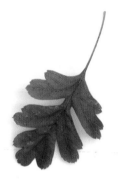

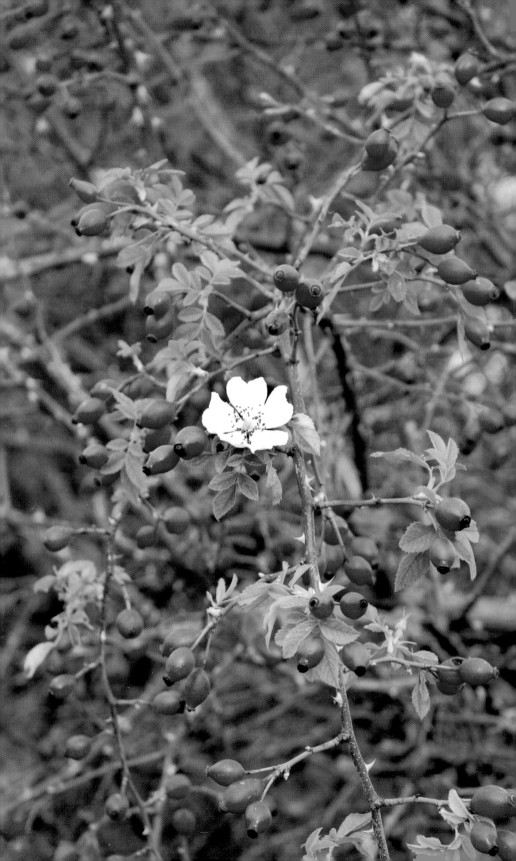

# BACKYARD
# MEDICINE

## Harvest and Make
## Your Own Herbal Remedies

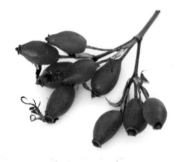

JULIE BRUTON-SEAL
MATTHEW SEAL

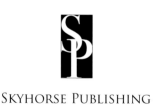

SKYHORSE PUBLISHING

Skyhorse Publishing books may be purchased in bulk at special discounts for sales promotion, corporate gifts, fund-raising, or educational purposes. Special editions can also be created to specifications. For details, contact the Special Sales Department, Skyhorse Publishing, 555 Eighth Avenue, Suite 903, New York, NY 10018 or info@skyhorsepublishing.com.

www.skyhorsepublishing.com

10 9 8 7 6 5 4 3 2 1

Library of Congress Cataloging-in-Publication Data

Bruton-Seal, Julie.
Backyard medicine : harvest and make your own herbal remedies / Julie Bruton-Seal & Matthew Seal.
p. cm.
Includes bibliographical references and index.
ISBN 978-1-60239-701-9 (alk. paper)
1. Herbs--Therapeutic use--Popular works. I. Seal, Matthew, 1946- II. Title.
RM666.H33B78 2008
615'.321--dc22
2008048431

Printed in China

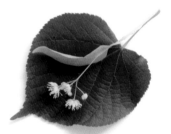

**Please note**:
The information in *Backyard Medicine* is compiled from a blend of historical and modern sources, from folklore and personal experience. It is not intended to replace the professional advice and care of a qualified herbal or medical practitioner. Do not attempt to self-diagnose or self-prescribe for serious long-term problems without first consulting a qualified professional. Heed the cautions given, and if already taking prescribed medicines or if you are pregnant, seek professional advice before using herbal remedies.

# Contents

Preface to the North American edition   vii
Preface to the British edition   vii
Introduction   ix
Harvesting from the wild   x
Using your herbal harvest   xii

Agrimony  2
Bilberry  6
Birch  12
Blackberry, Bramble  16
Burdock  20
Cherry  24
Chickweed  26
Cleavers  30
Coltsfoot  34
Comfrey  38
Couch grass  42
Curled dock, Yellow dock  46
Dandelion  50
Elder  56
Guelder rose, Crampbark  62
Hawthorn  64
Honeysuckle, Woodbine  70
Hops  72
Horse chestnut  74
Horseradish  78
Horsetail  80
Lime, Linden  84
Lycium  87
Mallow  92
Meadowsweet  96

Mint  100
Mugwort  104
Mullein  110
Nettle  114
Oak  120
Pellitory of the wall  124
Plantain  126
Ramsons, Bear garlic  132
Raspberry  136
Red clover  139
Red poppy  142
Rosebay willowherb, Fireweed  146
Self-heal  150
Shepherd's purse  155
St John's wort  158
Sweet cicely  164
Teasel  167
Vervain  170
White deadnettle  173
Wild lettuce  176
Wild rose  178
Willow  184
Willowherb  186
Wood betony  188
Yarrow  192

Notes to the text   198
Recommended reading   201
Resources   202
Index   203

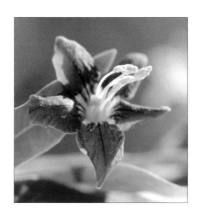

To our parents

Jen and Des Bartlett
Midge and George Seal

# Preface to the North American edition

We have taken the opportunity to correct the text and make the spelling more appropriate for North American readers. The substance of the book, however, remains as for the British edition. All the plants are found on both sides of the Atlantic, some being native in the New World and others brought over from Europe by settlers precisely because they were useful plants that they wanted to keep using.

We appreciate that some of the plants are less common in North America and that a few are classified as noxious or invasive (we give details of these in the text), but we believe that each of them is worth seeking out in the wild and has medicinal value. And if you do not have these plants growing near you, most of them can readily be grown in your own garden (subject to state or federal law).

In addition, the recipes we give can be adapted and used for other medicinal plants that may grow around you. We have made the measurements more North American-friendly by changing metric to standard, but the recipes remain simple and easy to follow.

Additional thanks go to Donna Bryant, David Hoffmann, Sara James, Maida Silverman, Karin Uphoff, and Matthew Wood.

As we write, the credit crunch and deepening recession are affecting all of us. But as the things of the money economy become scarcer, this is the time to look to our own backyards. We can grow more food and harvest our wild and cultivated plants for medicine. We can do so much for ourselves.

October 2008                                    Norfolk, UK

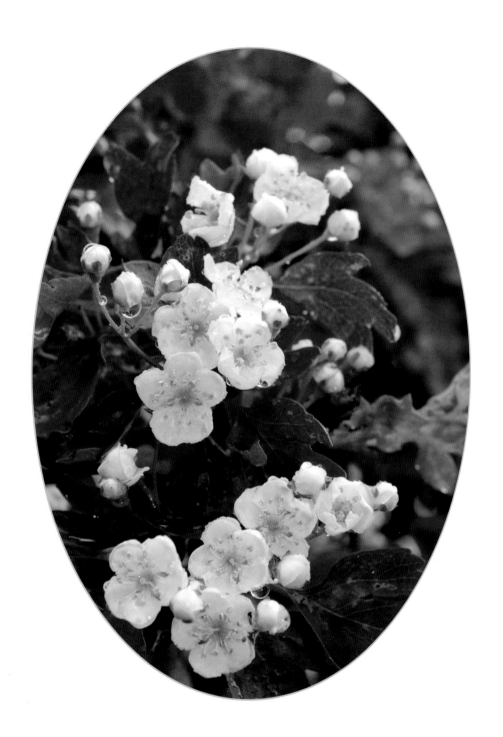

# Introduction

The British edition of this book used the title "hedgerow medicine," which we have changed to "backyard medicine" for the present edition.

Hedgerows in Britain are an integral part of the landscape, and the word conveys a sense of countryside and the often-forgotten traditional harvesting and use of plants – there are miles of public footpaths with rights of access. We wanted to suggest the same sense of self-sufficiency in using the plants that grow "on your doorstep," hence our choice of the term "backyard medicine."

The plants we have selected are found in various habitats, including both cultivated and neglected land. So do not be surprised to see pictures here of plants growing on cliff scree, a church wall, or open moorland. Quite a few of our plants are happy in cities, in waste lots, and parks, or cracks in sidewalks.

If we give ourselves some latitude in the first part of our title, what of "medicine"? Herbal medicines are traditional and effective, and we encourage you to use our chosen plants in making your own medicines. In the process you are taking responsibility for your own health. We do not intend to decry either pharmaceutical or manufactured herbal products, for clearly both have their place and many people want them. What we'd prefer to do is make a positive case for our wild plants.

Consider the following quotation from a 2004 survey of *Britain's Wild Harvest*, which is also relevant for the US. In terms of sourcing herbal medicines, it said that Britain is a major user of herbs, but "despite this interest our own wild species play a remarkably small role in this market. Almost all of the tinctures, creams or infusions we use derive from plants that we import or cultivate."

Using local plants for herbal remedies saves on imports and air miles; backyard medicines are not only cheap, they are free. There is also a sustainability issue: many popular imported herbal medicines have negative environmental effects in their place of origin. Our plants are common, local, often invasive plants written off or condemned as weeds.

An excellent reason to harvest and make your own local herbal medicines is the pleasure the whole process brings. You will also have the peace of mind of knowing exactly what is in your medicines. Then again, the current regulatory environment is running against over-the-counter herbal preparations, and there is almost certain to be less choice and more control in future. All in all, the best option is to learn to make your own remedies.

Do please be aware that this book is intended to be a general guide to plant medicines and is not specific to personal circumstances or meant to replace a professional consultation. Do not self-diagnose or self-treat for serious or long-term conditions without consulting a qualified herbal or medical practitioner.

Having said that, we hope to show you how easy it is to make your own remedies from wild plants. You will soon build up a home medicine cabinet better than anything you could buy. We support you in taking responsibility for your own health, and wish you well in seeking the healing virtues offered by the plants all around us.

# Harvesting from the wild

**Harvesting wild plants for food or medicine is a great pleasure, and healing in its own right. We all need the company of plants and wild places in our lives, whether this is in an old wood, a mountainside or the seashore, just down the street, or in our own backyard. Gathering herbs for free is the beginning of a valuable and therapeutic relationship with the wild. Here are a few basic guidelines to help you get started.**

*Why pay others to frolic in the luscious gardens of Earth, picking flowers and enjoying themselves making herbal products? You can do all that frolicking, immersing yourself in wondrous herbal beauty, and uplifting your mind and spirit. Making your own herbal medicine both enhances your happiness and boosts your immune system.*
– Green (2000)

When collecting, try to choose a place where the plant you are harvesting is abundant and vibrant. Woods, fields, and minor roads are best, though many of our fifty plants are also found in the city. Avoiding heavy traffic is safer for you and your lungs, and plants growing in quiet places are less polluted. Plants growing next to fields may receive crop sprays.

We usually want to harvest herbs when they are at their lushest. It's best to pick on a dry day, after the morning dew has burned off. For St John's wort and aromatic plants the energy of the sun is really important, so wait for a hot day and pick while the sun is high in the sky, ideally just before noon.

It is really important to make sure you have the right plant. A good field guide is essential – for North America we recommend the Peterson Field Guide series, which has regional guides including *A Field Guide to Medicinal Plants and Herbs of Eastern and Central North America*. Some herbalists and foragers offer herb walks – great for learning to identify plants. For distribution maps and other information, go to the USDA PLANTS database: http://plants.usda.gov/.

Harvest only what you need and will use; leave some of the plant so it will grow back. When picking "above-ground parts" of a plant, only take the top half to two-thirds. Never harvest a plant if it is the only one in a particular area.

We have included a few roots in our recipes. It is important not to over-harvest these, even though most of the plants we describe are widespread. The law states that you must seek the permission of the landowner before you dig up roots, if this is not on your own land (see p. 198 for more on law).

Collecting equipment is simple: think carrier bags or a basket, and perhaps gloves, scissors, or shears. If you are harvesting roots take a shovel or digging fork.

A quiet English country lane in May, with hawthorn flowering and a healthy undergrowth of nettles and cleavers.

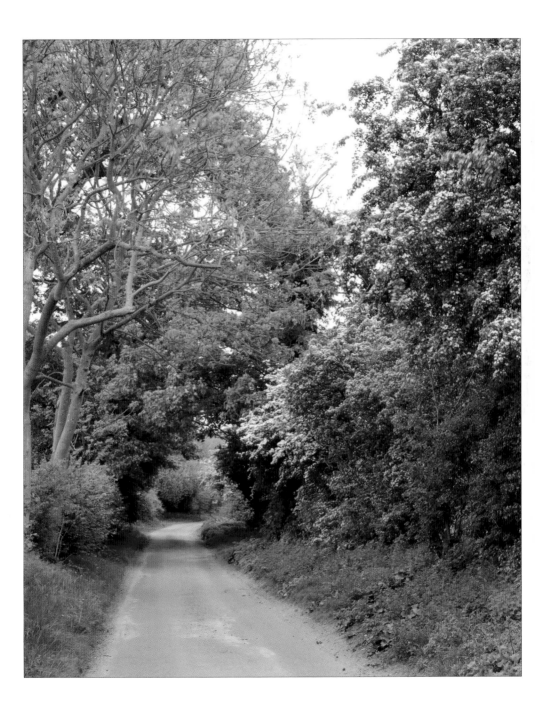

# Using your herbal harvest

**Herbs can be used in many different ways. Simplest of all is nibbling on the fresh plant, crushing the leaves to apply them as a poultice, or perhaps boiling up some leaves as a tea. Many of the plants discussed in this book are foods as well as medicines, and incorporating them seasonally in your diet is a tasty and enjoyable way to improve your health.**

**But because fresh herbs aren't available year round or may not grow right on your doorstep, you may want to preserve them for later use. Follow these guidelines.**

### Equipment needed
You don't need any special equipment for making your own herbal medicines. You probably already have most of what you need. Kitchen basics like a teapot, measuring cups, saucepans, and a blender are all useful, as are jam-making supplies such as a jelly bag and jam jars. A mortar and pestle are useful but not essential.

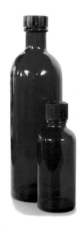

You'll need jars and bottles, and labels for these. It is a good idea to have a notebook to write down your experiences, so you'll have a record for yourself and can repeat successes. Who knows, it could become a future family heirloom like the stillroom books of old!

There is a list of suppliers at the end of the book to help you source any supplies or ingredients you may need.

### Drying herbs
The simplest way to preserve a plant is to dry it, and then use the dried part to make teas (infusions or decoctions). Dried plant material can also go into tinctures, infused oils, and other preparations, though these are often made directly from fresh plants.

To dry herbs, tie them in small bundles and hang these from the rafters or a laundry airer, or spread the herbs on a sheet of brown paper or a screen. (Avoid using newspaper as the inks contain toxic chemicals.) You can easily make your own drying screen by stapling some mosquito netting or other open-weave fabric to a wooden frame. This is ideal, as the air can circulate around the plant, and yet you won't lose any small flowers or leaves that are loose.

Generally, plants are best dried out of the sun. A linen cupboard works well, particularly in damp weather.

### Storing dried herbs
Once the plant is crisply dry, you can discard any larger stalks. Whole leaves and flowers will

keep best, but if they are large you may want to crumble them so they take up less space. They will be easier to measure for teas, etc. if they are crumbled before use.

Dried herbs can be stored in brown paper bags or in airtight containers such as candy jars or plastic tubs, in a cool place. If your container is made of clear glass or other transparent material, keep it in the dark as light will fade leaves and flowers quite quickly. Brown glass jars are excellent – we have happily worked our way through quantities of hot chocolate in order to build up a collection of these!

Dried herbs will usually keep for a year, until you can replace them with a fresh harvest. Roots and bark keep longer than leaves and flowers.

**Teas: infusions and decoctions**
The simplest way to make a plant extract is with hot water. Fresh or dried herbs can be used. An **infusion,** where hot water is poured over the herb and left to steep for several minutes, is the usual method for leaves and flowers.

A **decoction**, where the herb is simmered or boiled in water for some time, is needed for roots and

Part of a summer's herbal harvest: (*from left*) St John's wort in olive oil; dried mugwort; dandelion flower oil; raspberry vinegar; meadowsweet ghee; meadowsweet, mugwort, and mint in white wine; rosehip oxymel

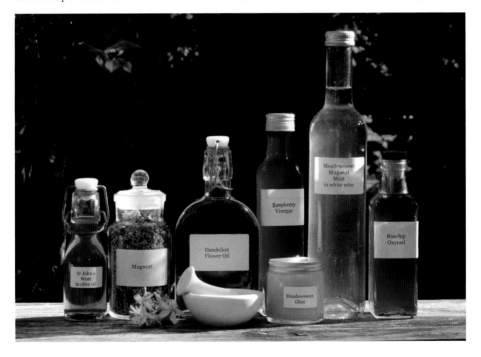

bark. Infusions and decoctions can also be used as mouthwashes, gargles, eyebaths, fomentations, and douches.

### Tinctures

While the term tincture can refer to any liquid extract of a plant, what is usually meant is an alcohol and water extract. Many plant constituents dissolve more easily in a mixture of alcohol and water than in pure water. There is the added advantage of the alcohol being a preservative, allowing the extract to be kept for several years.

The alcohol content of the finished extract needs to be at least 20% to adequately preserve it. Most commercially produced tinctures have a minimum alcohol content of 25%. A higher concentration is needed to extract more resinous substances, such as myrrh resin.

For making your own tinctures, vodka is the simplest alcohol as it can be used neat, has no flavor, and allows the taste of the herbs to come through. If you can get pure grain alcohol (95%) it can be diluted as needed. Whisky, brandy, or rum can also be used. Herbs can also be infused in wine, but this will not have as long a shelf life.

To make a tincture, you simply fill a jar with the herb and top up with alcohol, or you can put the whole lot in the blender first. It is then kept out of the light for anything from a day to a month to infuse before being strained and bottled.

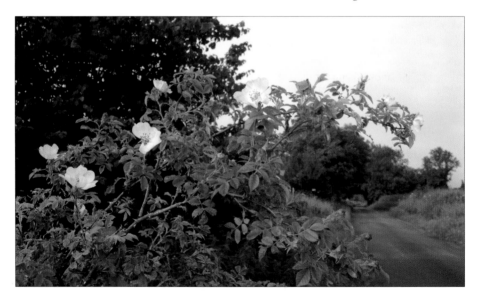

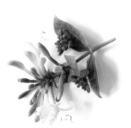

Tinctures are convenient to store and to take. We find amber or blue glass jars best for keeping, although clear bottles will let you enjoy the colors of your tinctures. Store them in a cool place. Kept properly, most tinctures have a shelf life of around five years. They are rapidly absorbed into the bloodstream, and alcohol makes the herbal preparation more heating and dispersing in its effect.

### Wines and beers

Many herbs can be brewed into wines and beers, which will retain the medicinal virtues of the plants. Elderberry wine and nettle beer are traditional examples, but don't forget that ordinary beer is brewed with hops, a medicinal plant.

### Glycerites

Vegetable glycerine is extracted from palm or other oil, and is a sweet, syrupy substance. It is particularly good in making medicines for children, and for soothing preparations intended for the throat and digestive tract, or coughs. A glycerite will keep well as long as the concentration of glycerine is at least 50% to 60% in the finished product.

Glycerine does not extract most plant constituents as well as alcohol does, but is effective for flowers such as red poppies, roses, and St John's wort. Glycerites are made the same way as tinctures, except the jar is kept in the sun or in a warm place to infuse.

Glycerine is a good preservative for fresh plant juices, in which half fresh plant juice and half glycerine are mixed, as it keeps the juice green and in suspension better than alcohol. This sort of preparation is called a **succus**.

### Vinegars

Another way to extract and preserve plant material is to use vinegar. Some plant constituents extract better in an acidic medium, making vinegar the perfect choice. Herbal vinegars are often made from pleasant-tasting herbs, and used in salad dressings and for cooking. They are also a good addition to the bath or for rinsing hair, as the acetic acid of the vinegar helps restore the natural protective acid pH of the body's exterior. Cider vinegar is a remedy for colds and other viruses, so it is a good solvent for herbs for these conditions.

### Herbal honeys

Honey has natural antibiotic and antiseptic properties, so is an excellent vehicle for medicines to fight infection. It can be applied topically to wounds and burns. Local honey can help prevent hayfever attacks.

Honey is naturally sweet, making it palatable for medicines for children. It is also particularly suited to medicines for the throat and respiratory system as it is soothing and also clears congestion. Herb-infused honeys are made the same way as glycerites, or can be gently heated in a bain-marie.

### Oxymels
An oxymel is a preparation of honey and vinegar. Oxymels were once popular as cordials, both in Middle Eastern and European traditions. They are particularly good for cold and flu remedies. Honey can be added to an herb-infused vinegar, or an infused honey can be used as well.

### Electuaries
These are made by stirring powdered dried herbs into honey or glycerine to make a paste. Electu-

aries are good as children's remedies, and are often used to soothe the digestive tract. This is also a good way to prepare tonic herbs.

### Syrups
Syrups are made by boiling the herb with sugar and water. The sugar acts as a preservative, and can help extract the plant material. Syrups generally keep well, especially the thicker ones containing more sugar, as long as they are stored in sterilized bottles.

They are particularly suitable for children because of their sweet taste, and are generally soothing.

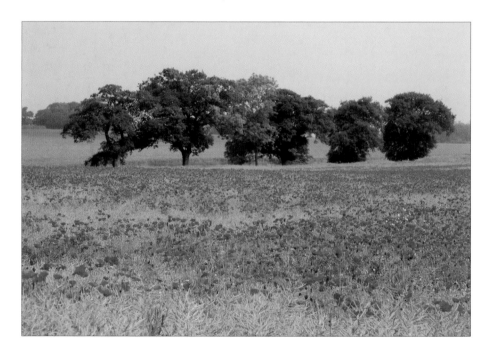

## Herbal sweets

While we are not recommending large amounts of sugar as being healthy, herbal sweets such as coltsfoot rock and peppermints are a traditional way of taking herbs in a pleasurable way.

## Plant essences

Plant essences, usually flower essences, differ from other herbal preparations in that they only contain the vibrational energy of the plant, and none of the plant chemistry. To make an essence, the flowers or other plant parts are usually put in water in a glass bowl and left to infuse in the sun for a couple of hours, as in the instructions for our self-heal essence. This essence is then preserved with brandy, and diluted for use.

## Infused oils

Oil is mostly used to extract plants for external use on the skin, but infused oils can equally well be taken internally. Like vinegars, they are good in salad dressings and in cooking.

We prefer extra virgin olive oil as a base, as it does not go rancid like many polyunsaturated oils do. Other oils, such as coconut and sesame, may be chosen because of their individual characteristics.

Infused oils are often called macerated oils, and should not be confused with essential oils, which are aromatic oils isolated by distilling the plant material.

## Ointments or salves

Ointments or salves are rubbed onto the skin. The simplest ointments are made by adding beeswax to an infused oil and heating until the beeswax has melted. The amount of wax needed will vary, depending on the climate or temperature in which it will be used, with more wax needed in hotter climates or weather.

Ointments made this way have a very good shelf life. They absorb well, while providing a protective layer on top of the skin.

Ointments can also be made with animal fats or hard plant fats such as cocoa butter.

## Butters and ghees

Butter can be used instead of oil to extract herbs, and, once clarified by simmering, it keeps well without refrigeration, making a simple ointment. Clarified butter is a staple in Indian cooking and medicine, where it is called ghee. It is soothing on the skin and absorbs well. Herbal butters and ghees can also be used as food.

## Skin creams

Creams are made by mixing a water-based preparation with an oil-based one, to make an emulsion. Creams are absorbed into the skin more rapidly than ointments, but have the disadvantages of being more difficult to make and not keeping as well. Essential oils can

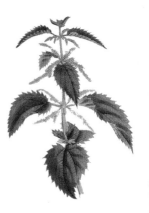

Nettle, from Woodville's *Medical Botany* (1790–3)

be added to help preserve creams, and they keep best if refrigerated.

### Poultices

The simplest poultice is mashed fresh herb put on to the skin, as when you crush a ribwort leaf and apply it to a wasp sting. Poultices can be made from fresh herb juice mixed with slippery elm powder or simply flour, or from dried herb moistened with hot water or vinegar.

Change the poultice every few hours and keep it in place with a bandage or bandaid.

### Fomentations or compresses

A fomentation or compress is an infusion or a decoction applied externally. Simply soak a flannel or bandage in the warm or cold liquid, and apply. Hot fomentations are used to disperse and clear, and are good for conditions as varied as backache, joint pain, boils, and acne. Hot fomentations need to be refreshed frequently once they cool down.

Cold fomentations can be used for inflammation or for headaches. Alternating hot and cold fomentations works well for sprains and other injuries.

### Embrocations or liniments

Embrocations or liniments are used in massage, with the herbs in an oil or alcohol base or a mixture of the two. Absorbed quickly through the skin, they can readily relieve muscle tension, pain, and inflammation, and speed the healing of injuries.

### Baths

Herbs can be added conveniently to bathwater by tying a sock or cloth full of dried or fresh herb to the hot tap as you run the bath, or by adding a few cups of an infusion or decoction. Herbal vinegars and oils can also be added to bath water, as can essential oils.

Besides full baths, hand and foot baths can be very effective, as can sitz or hip baths where only your bottom is in the water.

### Douches

Herbal infusions or decoctions can be used once they have cooled as douches for vaginal infections or inflammation.

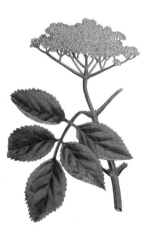

Elderflower, from Woodville's *Medical Botany* (1790–3); (opposite), elder in Lincolnshire, England in June

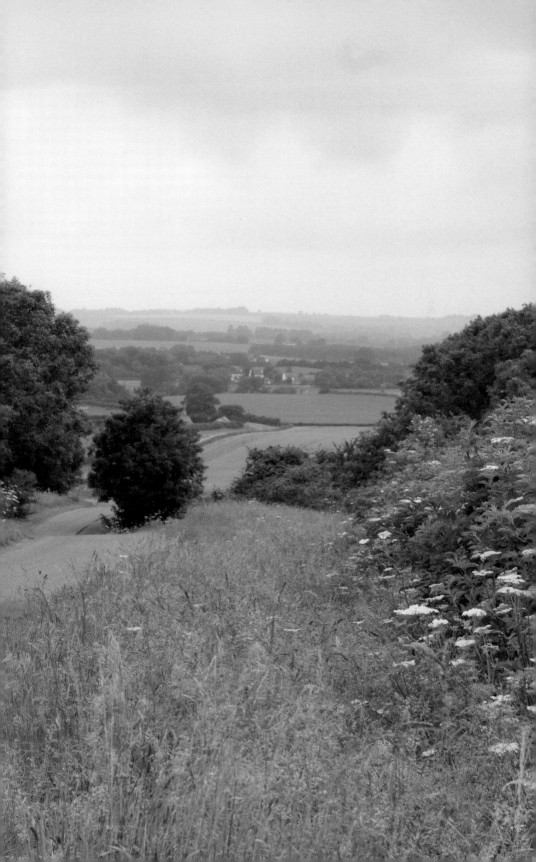

**Rosaceae**
**Rose family**

**Description:** Upright
perennials with spikes
of small yellow flowers
reaching up to 2 feet.

**Habitat:** Meadows
and roadsides/grassy
places.

**Distribution:** *A.
eupatoria* is native to
Europe and introduced
to North America. Tall
hairy agrimony, *A.
gryposepala*, is more
widespread and is used
interchangeably with
the European species.

**Related species:**
There are around
15 species of agri-
mony found in northern
temperate regions
and South America. In
China, *xian he cao* (*A.
pilosa*) is widely used
medicinally, mainly for
bleeding and diarrhea.
Cinquefoil and tormen-
til are old medicinal
herbs with very similar
properties to agrimony.

**Parts used:** Above-
ground parts, when in
flower in summer.

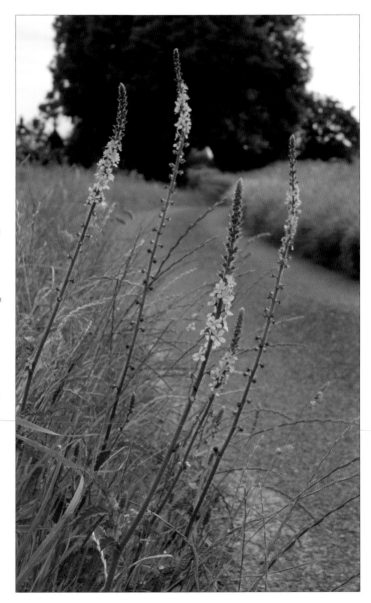

# Agrimony *Agrimonia eupatoria, A. procera, A. gryposepala*

**Agrimony stops bleeding of all sorts, and is used in trauma treatment and surgery in Chinese hospitals. It helps relieve pain too, and has a long tradition as a wound herb as well as for treating liver, digestive, and urinary tract problems.**

**Agrimony tightens and tones the tissues, and, in a seeming contradiction, also relaxes tension, both physical and mental. This is the herb for when you're feeling frazzled, when stress and tension or pain are causing torment.**

You can hardly miss this tall and bright summer garden herb, which readily earns its old name of church steeples. The sticky burrs that cling to passers-by lie behind another name, cocklebur.

Agrimony used to be a significant herb in the European tradition, being the Anglo-Saxon healing plant "garclive," but it is underused and underrated in modern western herbalism.

*Agrimonia eupatoria* is the "official" agrimony, but John Parkinson in *Theatrum Botanicum* (1640) preferred fragrant agrimony, *Agrimonia procera*, if available. The two can be used interchangeably.

In Chinese medicine, *A. pilosa* is the species used, and its name, *xian he cao*, translates as "immortal crane herb," which gives an idea of the reverence in which it is held. It is used in surgery and trauma treatment to stop bleeding, and has been found to be effective

against *Trichomonas* vaginal infections and tapeworms, as also for dysentery and chronic diarrhea.

Dr Edward Bach chose agrimony as one of his 38 flower essences. It is for people who soldier on, who say everything is fine when it is not, hiding inner turmoil behind a cheerful facade and ignoring the darker side of life. The out-of-balance agrimony person often resorts to alcohol, drugs, or adrenaline-producing sports to avoid dealing with life issues.

**Use agrimony for...**
Contemporary American herbalist Matthew Wood has written more deeply about agrimony than anybody else. He uses it as a flower essence, herbal tincture, and homeopathic preparation, and has researched it in great detail, expanding on the traditional picture of the plant. Wood calls agrimony "the bad hair day remedy" – imagine the cartoon picture

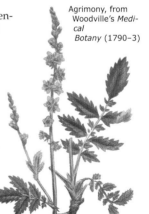

Agrimony, from Woodville's *Medical Botany* (1790–3)

**Agrimony tea**
• eyewash, conjunc-
tivitis
• gargle for mouth &
gum or throat problems
• in footbath for ath-
lete's foot
• in bath for sprains &
strained muscles

**Agrimony tincture**
• appendicitis
• urinary incontinence
• potty training
• cystitis
• weak digestion
• diarrhea/constipation
• tension
• irritable bladder
• asthma
• childhood diarrhea
• burns

*... there are few of our
wild flowers which are
in more esteem with
the village herbalist
than the agrimony.
Every gatherer of sim-
ples knows it well.*
– Pratt (1857)

healing to begin as blood and energy flow are brought back to normal.

Agrimony is a wonderful wound herb, as it rapidly stops bleeding and also relieves pain. It is thought that a high tannin and vitamin K content account for its remarkable coagulation properties. In the 1400s agrimony was picked to make "arquebusade water," to staunch bleeding inflicted by the arquebus or hand gun.

Agrimony works well for burns too – put tincture directly on the burn and take a few drops internally; repeat until pain subsides.

Agrimony has an affinity for the liver and digestive tract, working to co-ordinate their functions. John Parkinson – the herbalist to King James II and King Charles I – wrote in 1640 that "it openeth the obstructions of the Liver, and cleanseth it; it helpeth the jaundise, and strengthneth the inward parts, and is very beneficiall to the bowels, and healeth their inward woundings and bruises or hurts." All these are uses borne out today and explained by the herb's bitter and astringent qualities.

of a cat that has had a fright or put its paw into an electric socket. He has found it works for people with mental and physical tension or work-related stress, with "pain that makes them hold their breath" and a range of other conditions.

Agrimony is a great herb for treating intermittent fever and chills, or in alternating constipation and diarrhea, as it helps the body to recover a working balance between extremes, by releasing the tension and constricted energy that cause such problems.

Pain is very often associated with constriction, with one condition reinforcing the other. Agrimony can help release us from this self-perpetuating spiral, allowing body and mind to relax and restorative

Agrimony's other main affinity is for the urinary tract, being used to good effect to ease the pain of kidney stones, irritable bladder, and chronic cystitis. It can be given safely to children for bedwetting and anxiety about potty training, and to the elderly for incontinence.

### Harvesting agrimony

Harvest when the plant is in bloom in the summer, picking the flower spike and some leaves. For agrimony tea, dry them in the shade until crisp, and then strip the flowers and leaves off the stems, discarding the stems. Store in brown paper bags or glass jars, in a cool dry place.

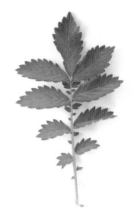

### Agrimony tea

Use 1–2 teaspoonfuls of **dried agrimony** per cup of **boiling water**, infused for 10 to 15 minutes. The tea has a pleasant taste and odor, and was often used as a country beverage, especially when imported tea was expensive.

**Dose:** The tea can be drunk three times a day, or used when cool as an eyewash or gargle for gum irritations and sore throats.

### Agrimony bath

Make a strong tea with a handful of **dried agrimony** infused in 1 pint of freshly **boiled water** for 20 minutes.

Poured hot into a foot bath, this soothes athlete's foot or sprained ankles; added to a hot bath it helps strained muscles after exercise, and general tension that has stiffened the muscles, back, and joints.

### Agrimony tincture

To make agrimony tincture, pick the **flowers and leaves** on a bright sunny day. Pack them into a glass jar large enough to hold your harvest – clean jam jars work well – and pour in enough **brandy or vodka** to cover them. Put the lid on the jar and keep it in a dark cupboard for six weeks, shaking it every few days. Strain off the liquid, bottle, and label.

Amber or blue glass bottles will protect your tincture from UV light. If you use clear glass bottles, you will need to keep your tincture in a dark cupboard. It doesn't need to be refrigerated and should keep for several years, although it is best to make a fresh batch every summer if you can.

**Dose:** For tension or interstitial cystitis: 3–5 drops in a little water three times a day; as an astringent to tone tissues (as in diarrhea), half a teaspoonful in water three times daily.

The tincture can be used as a first-aid remedy for burns. First cool the burn thoroughly by holding it under water running from the cold tap for several minutes. You can just pour a little tincture onto the burn, but for best results, wet a cotton ball with the tincture and hold it in place until the burn stops hurting.

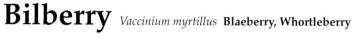

# Bilberry Vaccinium myrtillus **Blaeberry, Whortleberry**

**Bilberries are one of the best herbs for the eyes and eyesight. They also strengthen the veins and capillaries, so are used for fragile and varicose veins.**

**The leaves are healing too, being effective for urinary tract infections and helping to regulate blood sugar levels.**

**Ericaceae
Heather family**

**Description:** A short deciduous shrub with green twigs, pink flowers, and bluish-black berries.

**Habitat:** Heathland, moors, and woods with acid soils.

**Distribution:** Circumboreal in distribution, occurring in Europe, northern Asia, and in western North America.

**Related species:** North American blueberries are very similar to bilberries. There are several species, including highbush blueberry (*V. corymbosum*) and lowbush blueberry (*V. angustifolium*).

**Parts used:** Berries and leaves picked in summer.

Bilberry is an ancient source of food and medicine in northern Europe. Its long period of use is reflected in its many colorful British regional names: bilberry in northern England, blaeberry or blueberry in Scotland, wimberry in Shropshire, whortleberry in south-eastern England, and huckleberry in the Midlands.

In North America it grows wild in western states, and is known as European blueberry, whortleberry, or huckleberry. There are several similar North American species, including highbush blueberry (*V. corymbosum*), lowbush blueberry (*V. angustifolium*), and dwarf bilberry (*V. cespitosum*), that can be used the same way as bilberry, though not as well studied.

In Britain, gathering bilberries in high summer was once a regular family and social occasion, as well as a local cottage industry. The main food harvest, usually grain or potatoes, was about to begin, but the timing of early August was just right for a day celebrating bilberries.

Whether Fraughan Sunday in Ireland (from Gaelic for "that which grows in the heather"), whort or hurt day in southern England, Laa Luanya in the Isle of Man, and equivalent August picking days in Wales, Scotland, and the southwest, the pattern was similar.

Whole communities would visit hill tops, woods, lakes, or holy wells, and the more assiduous would pick bilberries in rush or willow baskets. This was a rare day out, and it was a noisy, happy, and often drunken occasion. It had predictable consequences, with unmarried boys and girls, off the leash for once, taking the chance to slip away and have more personal kinds of fun.

In Yorkshire, there was a more sober bilberry connection, with bilberry pies the traditional fare of funeral teas: berries mixed with sugar and lemon juice were baked in crusty pastry. Bilberry pies were known there as "mucky-mouth pies" because they stained your hands and mouth blue, though still deliciously worth the trouble.

Bilberry is a wild plant, rarely cultivated, and you must gather it for yourself if you want it. Picking bilberries takes the present-day forager as close to being a hunter-gatherer as one can get. For our ancestors, the harvest was more than recreational, it was an important source of nutrition.

Picking the berries is the perfect excuse to get out into wild nature, as bilberry grows on windswept moors or in heathy woodland. You have to get down to it on all fours to gather, especially on tundra and moors where the plants are very low-growing.

Harvesting the low-lying fruit was and is backaching work, but bilberries are so intensely flavor-ful and so loaded with nutritional benefits that it is still worth the effort today. Where commercial gathering was undertaken, as in Gwent, the process was sometimes eased by a toothed metal comb or rake, the *peigne*, named from a French tool, which could remove the berries from their stems. The fruit would be sold via dealers to jam-making factories, and sometimes for dyeing.

The dealers were reported as being annoyed in 1917 and 1918 when the bilberry crop was requisitioned for wartime dyeing needs and they made less on the deal than with the usual jam.

The berries made more than jam, going into wine and liqueurs in

**Anthocyanins**
These are a class of flavonoid compounds, found in high levels in bilberries. Anthocyanins are pigments that give red or blue color to blackberries, elderberries, hawthorn berries, cherries, and many other fruits and vegetables. These compounds are powerful antioxidants that are attracting a lot of attention in nutritional research. Their potential health benefits include easing the effects of aging, reducing inflammation and increasing insulin production. Anthocyanins also protect the blood vessels and have a range of anti-cancer effects.

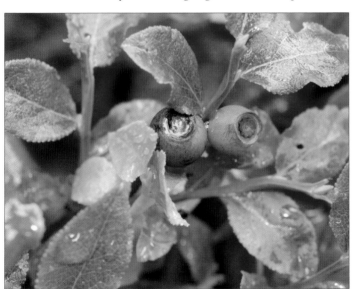

*It is a pity they [bilberries] are used no more in physic than they are.*
– Culpeper (1653)

*… the first and most indispensable of all the tinctures in our family medicine chest.*
– Abbé Kneipp (1821–97), on fresh bilberry tincture

Scotland and on the Continent. As well as a purple dye, in medieval times the bilberry was also tried as a writing ink and paint. Sources of purply-blue paint became increasingly important in the Middle Ages as coloring in depictions of the Virgin Mary's gown.

Bilberries have always been found nutritious and safe to eat fresh; also they are not spiny and only have small internal pips. They are equally good dried for later use in the home or while traveling. However, they are so delicious eaten straight off the bush or fresh with a little cream that you may never have any left to preserve.

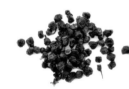

Bilberries have remained a favorite for their sweet, deep-toned, and slightly astringent flavor in pies, jams, and syrups. Commercial jam-makers appreciated them because they have fewer seeds than most other soft fruits and also more pectin. This meant that less sugar was needed to set them, one pound of sugar setting two pounds of fruit (other fruit recipes usually specify about equal amounts of fruit and sugar). No wonder bilberry made a cheap and popular jam, one also rich in vitamins C and A, and healthier because it had less sugar.

### Use bilberry for…

There's an interesting story about bilberry jam that neatly links its commercial and medicinal uses. Back in the early days of the Second World War, British pilots going on night missions chanced on

the fact that eating bilberry jam sandwiches before flying would improve their nightsight. This all might seem "jolly prang" apocryphal, but research has confirmed that taking bilberry stimulates production of retinal purple, known to be integral to night vision.

The berry's eyesight benefits are now recognized as also including treatment of glaucoma, cataracts and general eye fatigue. Bilberry seems to work by its tonic effect on the small blood vessels of the eye, thereby improving the micro-circulation.

So taking bilberry as a tea, syrup, wine, dried fruit, jelly, or jam is officially good for eyes as well as your taste buds!

This is a relatively new feature of bilberry's repertoire. Mrs Grieve, the modern standard among British herbals, published in 1931, doesn't mention taking bilberry for eyesight. But, as you come to expect from reading Mrs Grieve, she is thorough on historical uses.

So she mentions that the berries, being diuretic, antibacterial, and disinfectant, as well as mildly astringent, are an old remedy for diarrhea, dysentery, gastroenteritis, and the like. A bilberry syrup was traditionally made in Scotland for diarrhea. Eating a handful of the dried berries works well too.

The berry tea was used for treating bedwetting in children, and to dilate blood vessels of the body, in the same way as described for the eye. The tea is valuable for varicose veins and hemorrhoids, strengthening vein and capillary walls. The berries mashed into a paste are applied to hemorrhoids.

Then there are the bilberry leaves, which are a valuable herbal medicine in their own right, with a slightly different range of qualities, although often used in combination with the berries. The leaves are deciduous, and turn a beautiful red in autumn before they fall.

The particular and long-appreciated effect of the leaves is as an antiseptic tea for treating urogenital tract inflammation, especially of the bladder. This tea can also be drunk for ulcers, including of the mouth and tonsils.

Bilberry leaves are known to be hypoglycemic, i.e., they reduce blood sugar levels, and are used successfully in treating late-onset diabetes. This is a slow-acting treatment, however, and taking the tea for long periods may lead to a build-up of tannins that is counter-productive. Some sources suggest using the leaf tea for only three weeks at a time; others say it is best with strawberry leaves.

Julie uses bilberry syrup for eyesight and vascular problems. She says:

"A friend once asked me to make up bilberry syrup for her elderly

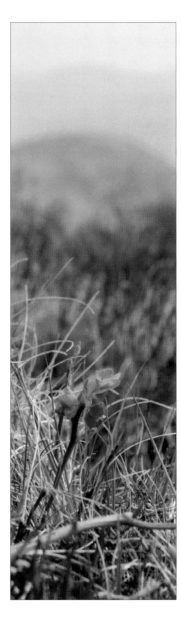

*Many a lad met his wife on Blaeberry Sunday.* – traditional Irish saying

*This fruit and its relatives ... have been used traditionally for problems with visual acuity. And scientific research has validated this folk medicine approach.* – Duke (1997)

Bilberry flowers on the Long Mynd, Shropshire, England in April

neighbor. This lady had a lot of aching and discomfort in her legs from varicose veins but was about to go on a long walk, the pilgrimage to Santiago de Compostela in Spain. She completed the pilgrimage successfully, walking many miles, commenting that she could 'feel her veins tightening up' when she took the syrup."

Bilberry combines well with ginkgo tincture or glycerite for eye problems. Julie's father has been taking this combination ever since he had surgery for a detached retina many years ago. His eye surgeon was initially sceptical, but checked into the research and now regularly recommends both these herbs to his patients.

Julie has used this combination for macular degeneration or retinal tears. Two cases stand out, both people with small tears in the retina. These were not bad enough to warrant surgery, but were intensely worrying to the people concerned, who came to see her to learn if further damage could be prevented.

In both cases, the patients went back to their eye specialists after taking bilberry and ginkgo for several months, and the specialists said words to the effect of "but there's nothing there, we must have made a mistake when we looked at your eyes initially." Not everyone may be as fortunate, but bilberry certainly has an important role to play in promoting and restoring eye health.

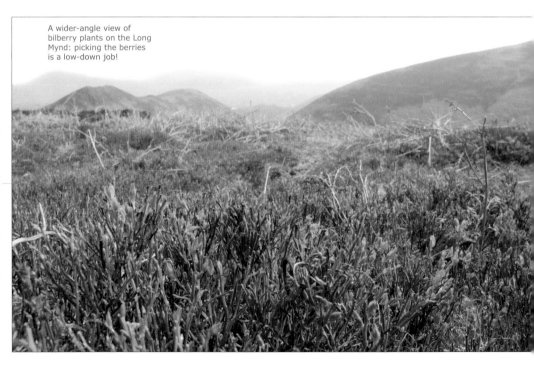

A wider-angle view of bilberry plants on the Long Mynd: picking the berries is a low-down job!

### Bilberry syrup

Place your **bilberries** in a saucepan with just enough **water** to cover them. Simmer gently for half an hour, then leave to cool before squeezing out as much of the liquid as possible using a jelly bag. For every pint of liquid, add 1 pound **demerara sugar**, and boil until the sugar has dissolved completely. Pour into sterile bottles, label, and store in a cool place.

**Dose:** 1 teaspoonful daily to maintain good eyesight and vascular health. For more acute problems, take 1 teaspoonful three times daily.

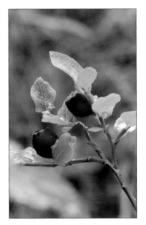

**BILBERRY BERRY**

**Syrup or glycerite**
- macular degeneration
- detached retina
- night vision
- cataracts
- capillary fragility

### Bilberry glycerite

Fill a jar with **bilberries** and pour on **vegetable glycerine** to take up all the air spaces. Put the lid on and shake to get rid of any remaining bubbles, then top up again with glycerine. Keep the jar in a warm place, such as on a sunny windowsill or by a wood stove, for two or three weeks, then squeeze out the liquid using a jelly bag. Bottle, label, and store in a cool place.

**Dose:** 1 teaspoonful daily to maintain good eyesight and vascular health. For more acute problems, take 1 teaspoonful three times daily.

### Berry brandy pot

Start out with **bilberries**, placing them in the bottom of a jar or crock and then pouring on enough **brandy (or whisky)** to cover. You can, of course fill the whole jar with bilberries, or you can leave room and repeat the process with **other berries** in layers as they come into season – raspberries, blackberries, elderberries, and lycium berries. Leave until winter and enjoy as a rather alcoholic treat, which will be packed with antioxidants and do your eyes and your veins a world of good. The liquid can be poured off and added to your syrup or glycerite, or left and enjoyed with the berries as a dessert with cream or however you like them.

### Bilberry leaf tea

Use a heaped teaspoonful of the **dried leaves** per cup or mug of **boiling water** and leave to infuse for 5 to 10 minutes.

**Dose:** Drink a cupful every few hours for an acute urinary infection, or one cup daily to help maintain blood sugar levels.

**BILBERRY LEAF**

**Bilberry leaf tea**
- urinary tract infections
- high blood sugar

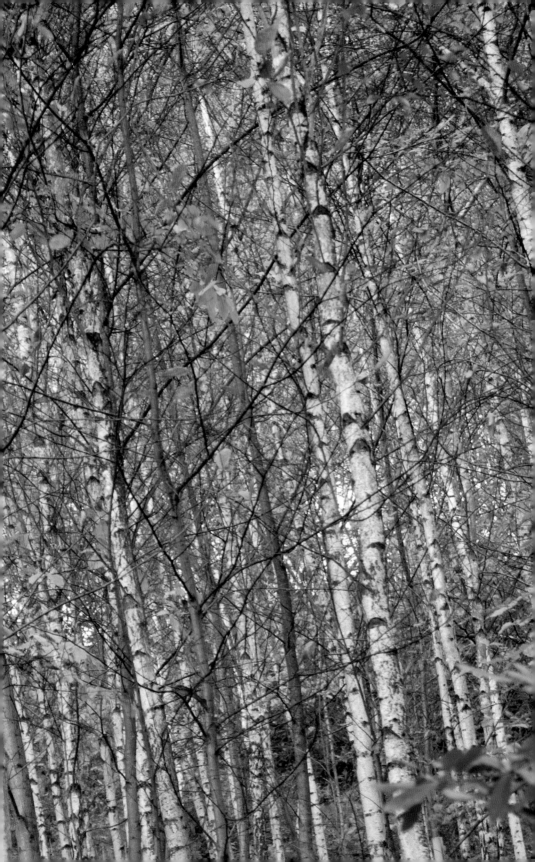

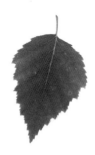

# Birch _Betula pendula, B. pubescens, B. lenta_

**Birch has a multitude of historical uses but is less familiar for its undoubted medicinal benefits. The sap makes a clear and refreshing drink that can be preserved as a wine, beer, or spirit. The leaves produce a pleasant tea and an infused oil. In each form, birch is an excellent tonic and detoxifier, mainly working on the urinary system to remove waste products, as in kidney or bladder stone, gravel, gout, and rheumatism. It reduces fluid retention and swellings, and clears up many skin problems.**

Birch is one of the most useful of trees as well as one of the most graceful. From adhesives to wine, baskets to yokes, and boats to vinegar, it has been a boon to people in the cold north for thousands of years. Its medicinal qualities have been historically valued and should be better known today.

Called the oldest tree in Britain, birch was a pioneer species when the ice caps retreated, moving in on the devastated land, growing quickly and then rotting to leave more fertile earth in which other species could take over. In its rapid life cycle birch pushes upward too fast to develop a strong heart wood, but this makes it perfect for making buckets and canoes.

As a youngster (writes Matthew), I was a suburban Hiawatha, and wanted to be a "Red Indian." I had read in my weekly comic, the

_Eagle_, how my heroes had made birch bark canoes and wrote on bark paper. Birch was a common enough tree, but I never really got down to the canoe or the paper. Soccer was more important.

But now these memories return, as Julie and I tap a birch in our garden. It is that time in spring after most of the frosts and before the birch buds and leaves emerge. The tree is now forcing its sap upward in prodigious quantity, and you simply tap into the flow, remembering to be kind to the tree after you have taken your share by closing off the wound.

Birch sap is rich in fructose whereas maple has sucrose. Sucrose is sweeter to the taste and the maple yields more per tree, so maple syrup is by far the bigger commercial industry. On the other hand, birch sap is cool, refreshing and clear. It tastes even better when reduced by simmering down into a golden-brown ambrosia. It's the sort of drink the elves would envy!

A stand of silver birch in the English Surrey hills, where the birch is so common it earned the name "Surrey weed"

**Betulaceae
Birch family**

**Description:** Deciduous trees that often hybridize, with whitish papery bark.

**Habitat:** Woods, heaths, moors, and gardens. Downy birch prefers wetter places.

**Distribution:** Silver birch or European white birch (_Betula pendula_) and downy birch (_B. pubescens_) are native to northern temperate regions of Eurasia, and found as introduced species in North America. Sweet birch (_B. lenta_) is native to eastern North America.

**Related species:** Worldwide, several birch species have medicinal value. In Ayurveda, Himalayan silver birch (_B. utilis_) is used.

**Parts used:** Sap, tapped in early spring; leaves, gathered in spring and early summer. The bark is also used.

## Use birch for...

Birch sap, birch water, or blood, had a folk reputation for breaking kidney or bladder stone and treating skin conditions and rheumatic diseases. It can be drunk in spring as a refreshing and cleansing tonic, clearing the sluggishness of winter from the system. The fermented sap also makes birch wine and country beers and spirits.

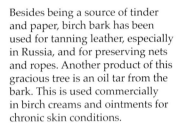

Besides being a source of tinder and paper, birch bark has been used for tanning leather, especially in Russia, and for preserving nets and ropes. Another product of this gracious tree is an oil tar from the bark. This is used commercially in birch creams and ointments for chronic skin conditions.

The fresh leaves or buds of birch offer a powerful but pleasant tea for general detoxing, urinary complaints, cystitis, rheumatic and arthritic troubles, and gout. Some herbalists add a pinch of sodium bicarbonate to improve the tea's ability to cut high uric acid levels. Any condition of fluid retention, such as cardiac or renal edema and dropsy, will be helped by the tea. Birch is rich in potassium, so that (like dandelion) it does not deplete the body of this mineral in the way that medical diuretics do.

Being such a good eliminator, birch tea is also effective as a compress applied directly to the skin for herpes, eczema, and the like.

You can easily make your own birch leaf oil by infusing the leaves in olive or sweet almond oil. This goes into commercial cellulite treatments, and can be used as a massage oil to relieve muscle aches and pains, fibromyalgia, and rheumatism. Drink birch tea as well for maximum benefit.

Birch is regarded as safe medicinally and no side effects have been reported.

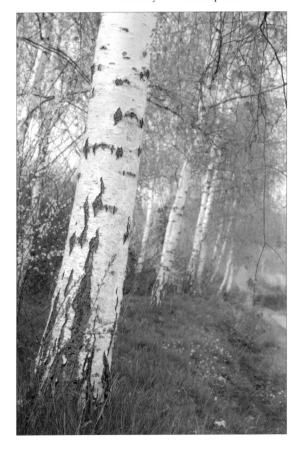

## Birch leaf oil

Pick the **leaves** in late spring or early summer, while they are still fresh and light green. Put them in a jar large enough to hold them and pour in enough **extra virgin olive oil or sweet almond oil** to cover them. Put a piece of cloth over the jar as a lid, held on with a rubber band. This will allow any moisture released by the leaves to escape. Put the jar in a sunny place indoors and leave for a month but stir it fairly regularly, checking to see that the leaves are kept beneath the surface of the oil.

Strain off into a jug, using a nylon jelly bag or a large strainer (if you use muslin, it will soak up too much of the oil). Allow to settle – if there is any water in the oil from the leaves, it will sink to the bottom of the jug. Pour the oil into sterile storage bottles, leaving any watery residue behind in the jug, and label. Using amber, blue, or green glass will protect the oil from ultraviolet light, so if you use clear glass bottles remember to store your oil away from light.

This can be used as a massage oil for cellulite, fibromyalgia, rheumatism, and other muscle aches and pains. It can be also used on eczema and psoriasis – but remember that these also need to be treated internally, so ask your herbalist for advice.

## Birch leaf tea

Pick the leaves in spring and early summer while they are still a fresh bright green. They can be used fresh in season or dried for later use. To dry, spread the leaves on a sheet of paper or on a drying screen, which can be made by stretching and stapling a piece of netting to a wooden frame. Dry them in the shade, until crisp when crumbled.

To make the tea, use 4 or 5 **leaves** per cup or mug of **boiling water,** and allow to infuse for 5 to 10 minutes.

**Dose:** Drink a cupful up to three or four times daily.

## Birch sap

To collect the sap, drill a hole through the bark in the early spring, before the tree gets its leaves. Insert a tube into the hole – a straw with a flexible end works well – and put the other end in a bottle or collection bucket. After you have collected for about a week, make sure you plug the hole with a twig the right size so that the tree doesn't keep "bleeding."

The sap is a delightfully refreshing drink as it comes from the tree, or it can be gently simmered down to taste to produce an amber ambrosia or further reduced to make a syrup.

**Birch leaf oil**
- cellulite
- detoxing massage
- aching muscles
- rheumatism
- eczema
- psoriasis

**Birch leaf tea**
- spring cleanse
- kidney stones
- urinary gravel
- cystitis
- gout
- arthritis
- rheumatism
- psoriasis
- eczema
- fluid retention
- fevers

**Birch sap**
- cleansing tonic

Our own crude birch tap: you can probably do better!

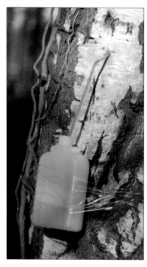

# Blackberry, Bramble *Rubus fruticosus*

**Rosaceae**
**Rose family**

**Description:** A thorny, sprawling bush with white or pink flowers and black berries.

**Habitat:** Widespread in hedgerows, woods, and on waste ground.

**Distribution:** Widespread. Native to temperate Europe but naturalized in North America and Australasia.

**Related species:** Blackberry is actually an aggregate of many taxonomically challenging species. It is related to dewberry (*R. caesius*), which has fruits with fewer, large segments and a blue bloom, and raspberry (*R. idaeus*).

**Parts used:** Leaves, gathered in early summer, berries harvested when ripe.

**Blackberry or bramble is one of the most familiar and also most aggressive of berry plants. The protective spines demand respect, but the berries and leaves offer medicinal rewards that repay the inevitable scratches of picking.**

The poet Walt Whitman wrote this about blackberry in "Song of Myself" (1855):

*I believe a leaf of grass is no less than the journey work of the stars/ ... and the running blackberry would adorn the parlors of heaven.*

In more sober judgment, Jonathan Roberts's history of fruit and vegetables (2001) calls blackberry a "primitive thug." Sorry to say, Roberts is probably closer to the truth. Blackberry always has been an aggressive settler on waste or cleared land, using an array of effective spreading mechanisms.

It is promiscuous in hybridizing with similar thorny trailing plants of the rose family (over 2,000 blackberry "species" have been described in Europe); then, it has tasty berries to spread its seeds, which pass unharmed through birds and humans alike; its young shoots bend to the ground and start fresh roots; its thorns hook on to adjacent foliage and help spread

the plant laterally; and its dense ground cover shuts off most competing plants.

The old ironic name of "lawyers" for blackberries has been exported from England to the United States: in either case, once in their clutches you will never escape! (Perhaps the makers of the handheld wireless device of the same name hoped for the same sense of being captured by their product.)

Highlanders in Scotland had a high opinion of blackberry. Its Gaelic name was *an druise bennaichte*, meaning "blessed bramble." This referred to Jesus supposedly using a bramble switch when riding his donkey to Jerusalem to evict the moneylenders from the temple. Highlanders made wreaths of ivy, bramble, and rowan as protection against evil.

Blackberry has been spread from the temperate north around the world apart from the tropics. New Zealand has become overrun to

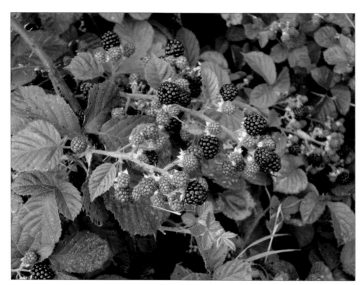

Blackberries are the most commonly used natural fruit in Great Britain. ... The fruit, so beloved of wine and jam makers, has rich medicinal properties, full of vitamin C and minerals, as are the leaves.
– Furnell (1985)

such an extent that there is a saying: there are only two brambles in New Zealand, one covering North Island and one South Island. In Australia it is a notifiable pest that must be destroyed wherever found; over 9 million hectares of land have been infested.

Blackberry hedges were used as defensive barriers around Native American settlements and in bygone Europe. Hedgerows containing blackberries make fields stock-proof, which is another reason why they are so widespread.

Sleeping Beauty, in the legend, was protected for a hundred years by a thicket of blackberry or perhaps wild rose – either would have been impenetrable after even two years by any but a true lover!

Going blackberrying or brambling is an ancient social activity worldwide, and family expeditions to gather the delicious fruit are well within living memory, though happening less in Britain these days. In the Ozark mountains, where communal picking still goes on, the bramble harvest is called "black gold."

Perhaps because blackberry was and still is so successful in the wild it was only in the nineteenth century that it was grown as a commercial crop, in the United States. It was also in the States that Judge Logan developed a cross raspberry/blackberry, named the loganberry in his honor. The friendlier raspberry meanwhile had been domesticated in Britain by the sixteenth century.

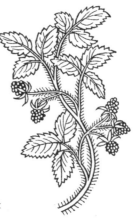

A medieval illustration of blackberry

We recommend you revive or continue the wild-picking habit because blackberries are so good for you and can be found almost everywhere. The ripe black fruit, as everyone knows, makes wonderful jams, jellies, preserves, pies, and cordials. The wine even stars in its own novel (*Blackberry Wine*, by Joanne Harris). But folklore dictates that you should not gather the berries after Michaelmas, because that is when the Devil spits or urinates on them. Or, we'd now say, the frost has got to them.

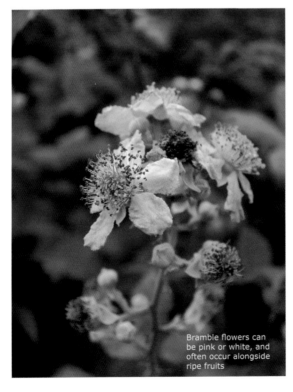

Bramble flowers can be pink or white, and often occur alongside ripe fruits

**Use blackberry for...**

In spring, blackberry shoots and the young leaves are a traditional European tonic, packed with vitamins and minerals, and used fresh as a tea. They can also be combined with raspberry leaves, young hawthorn leaves, and birch shoots or leaves.

The leaves and unripe fruit are good medicine too, for their astringency. In some places the leaves were chewed to allay headaches. Crushed blackberry leaves are exactly what you need as a styptic to treat small wounds or cuts incurred when picking the fruit; they also work for boils and swellings.

The main use of the leaf tea is as a folk remedy for diarrhea; the unripe red or green fruit can be used for the same purpose.

In the US Civil War of 1861–65 the ferocious hand-to-hand fighting in the woods was sometimes interrupted for "blackberry truces." Both sides would take time out to pick blackberry leaves for a tea to treat diarrhea and dysentery, which were rife in both armies.

The leaf tea is like a green tea, pleasant but with a tannin feel. It is also a welcome relief for problems of the mouth, such as ulcers and gum disease. It was once thought to strengthen teeth, and is an old remedy for soothing sore throats and treating colds and anemia. When cool, the tea makes a good skin lotion.

### Bramble leaf tea

Bramble leaves should be picked in spring and summer while they are fresh and green. They can be used fresh for tea in season, or can be dried for the winter. Dry them in a shady place or indoors, until the leaves are brittle and crumble easily. Store in brown paper bags or in jars in a cool, dark place.

To make the tea, put a few **fresh leaves** or a rounded teaspoonful of crumbled **dry leaves** in a teapot. Pour on a mugful of **boiling water**, and allow to infuse for about 5 minutes, then strain and drink.

**Dose:** Can be drunk freely. Make double-strength to treat diarrhea, drinking a cupful every hour as needed.

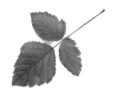

**Bramble leaf tea**
- general health
- diarrhea
- mouth ulcers
- gingivitis
- sore throats
- colds
- flu and fevers

### Blackberry spread

This is a traditional recipe, sometimes called "blackberry butter," which is delicious with scones or on toast.

Put in a pan: **1 pound blackberries**
**1 pound tart apples, chopped up but not peeled or cored**
**grated zest and juice of a lemon**

Simmer gently for about 15 minutes, until soft and mushy. Rub the pulp through a sieve to remove the skins and pips. Weigh the pulp, and for every 4oz of pulp add 3oz of **sugar**.

Heat gently until the sugar has dissolved, then simmer and stir until the mixture is thick and smooth – this usually takes about 20 minutes. Pour into sterilized jars, seal, and label.

### Blackberry oxymel

Pick blackberries when they are ripe, checking that the heel, the place where they come off the stem, is white or pale green – if this has gone purple or dark, it's not a good one to use.

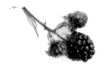

**Blackberry oxymel**
- general health
- colds
- sore throats

Put the **blackberries** in a china or glass bowl and pour on enough **white wine vinegar** just to cover them. Put a plate or a cloth over the bowl and leave it for a day or two, then crush the fruit with a potato masher. Strain the juice through a sieve or jelly bag into a measuring jug, then pour into a saucepan. Add half the volume of **honey,** then heat to melt the honey. Bring to a boil and boil for 5 minutes, bottle and label. This syrup can also be frozen in an ice cube tray, and then stored in bags in the freezer.

**To use:** Mix one tablespoonful with a cup of hot water as a bedtime drink, or drink frequently to help relieve a cold.

# Burdock *Arctium* spp.

**Asteraceae (Compositae) Daisy family**

**Description:** A biennial plant with large, soft, light green leaves and thistle-like red-purple flowers that form burrs with hooked spines. Can reach a sculptural 6 feet tall in its second year.

**Habitat:** Hedgerows, wood edges, and waste ground.

**Distribution:** Native to Europe and Asia, but found in temperate regions around the world; taken to North America by European settlers.

**Species used:** Greater or common burdock (*Arctium lappa*) is the best-known species, but lesser burdock (*A. minus*) is more widespread. It is similar in appearance and used interchangeably for medicinal purposes.

**Parts used:** Leaves picked in summer, roots dug in spring or fall, and seeds gathered in fall

**Traditionally combined with dandelion both as a soft drink and a medicine, burdock is a powerful cleanser and blood purifier. It is one of the foremost detoxing herbs, and is particularly effective for skin problems. The root is a food as well as a medicine, and is popular in Japanese cooking.**

Burdock is a sturdy biennial, with a rosette of large leaves forming in the first year, as the tap root deepens. In the second year the stems shoot up, producing the thistle-like flowers or burrs that gave it the old name of beggar's buttons.

The roots are best used in the first fall or second spring, and are more tonic in the spring. Descending nearly a yard, the mature root takes energetic digging up, but younger roots are just as good.

Burdock can be grown in the garden (one has adopted us, and we are happy to host it), and if you use raised beds or drainage pipes the root is much less effort to harvest. The other advantage is that you will know where to dig for spring roots, as the leaves die back to very little in the winter and the plants can be difficult to find.

Burdock root was a food for our hunter-gatherer ancestors, and is appreciated as a cooked vegetable in Japan, *gobo*; the dish is now popular in Hawaii and New Zealand. Its delicious mild flavor is similar to artichoke or scorzonera. Burdock is often called the velcro plant. This all comes from walking the dog: Swiss inventor George de Mestral noticed that after he and his dog had brushed by a large burdock, the plant's "hooks" had tagged onto "loops" in his wool trousers and in the dog's fur.

Using the technique of "biomimicry," De Mestral made two nylon pads, one of hooks and one of loops; the more you pushed them, the more they fused, but they pulled apart easily, just like the plant's fruits do in nature.

As NASA later used his Velcro™-derived products for astronaut suits, burdock (by proxy) became the first space weed. It's the latest version of a story played out over the centuries, with immigrants' clothes and their livestock fur transferring the benefits and burdens of burdock across the seas to new lands.

In terms of the British soft drink, a few specialist makers still use real roots in their dandelion and burdock mix but the mass market version has artificial flavorings.

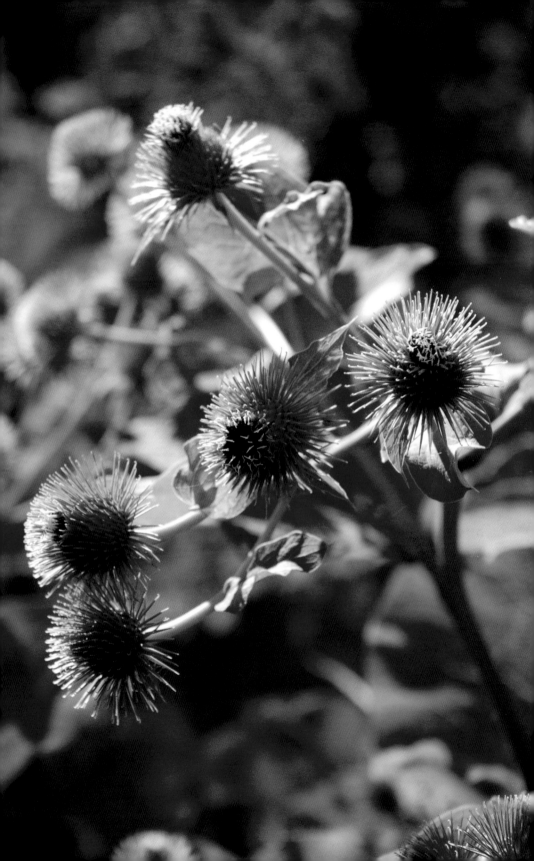

*Burdock is a "deep food" and alterative that moves the body to a state of well-nourished health, promotes the healing of wounds, and removes the indicators of system imbalance such as low energy, ulcers, skin conditions, and dandruff.*
– Green (2000)

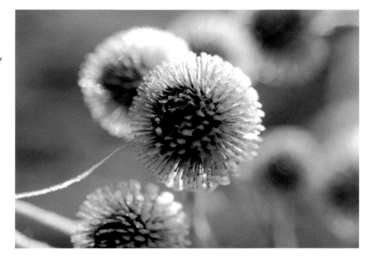

## Use burdock for...

Burdock is a significant detoxing herb in both Western and Chinese medicinal traditions. Known as a blood purifier, its special attribute is to stimulate the release of waste products from the cells. This is a powerful process at cellular level, and the metabolic wastes then need to be removed from the body.

Here is where the dandelion comes in, making a wonderful complement to burdock with its diuretic and flushing qualities to the outside world via the kidneys and liver. Hence the classic mix of the two roots. Burdock also combines well with red clover or dock.

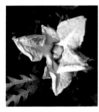

Burdock leaves emerging in early spring of the second year.

Herbal blood purifiers have the associated virtue of cleansing the skin. Burdock is known for its remarkable effect on skin conditions arising from imbalance, as in dry or scaly skin, and eruptions, as in acne, boils, eczema, and psoriasis. It can be applied externally as a poultice in addition to taking it internally as a decoction or tincture.

Burdock helps restore and maintain fluid balance in the body, both of water and of fats.

In the past burdock was associated with medical conditions that seemed incurable, if not evil, at the time. Mixed with wine in the Middle Ages, it was given for leprosy; later it was used to treat syphilis (Henry VIII improved, but was not cured by it), epilepsy, and hysteria; in modern times research has suggested possible benefits in treating HIV and cancer. Hildegard of Bingen was already using burdock root on her cancer patients in the 1100s. In each case burdock strongly supported the immune system.

Burdock root is used to break down excess uric acid in the joints that leads to gout. It also relieves arthritis and swollen prostate. Ask your herbalist's advice on the best combination of herbs for your own condition and constitution.

Another burdock benefit lies in its bitterness, which helps stimulate the digestive fluids and promote appetite and digestion. This underlies the tang of the famous drink and makes burdock palatable in anorexia.

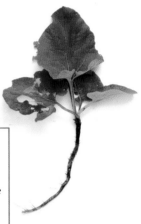

### Burdock leaf poultice

A simple poultice can be made from a whole burdock leaf. Steam it to soften the leaf, and apply as hot as can be borne to the affected place. Leave it there until it cools down and then heat again, or put a hot water bottle over it to keep it warm, and leave on for half an hour. The poultice will draw blood to the area, and as it is also antiseptic it will fight infection and accelerate healing.The leaves can also be crushed with a rolling pin and applied as a poultice for minor burns; leave them in place until the pain subsides.

### Harvesting burdock root

As burdock is a biennial, the roots need to be dug at the end of the first year or in early spring of the second year. The plant then puts all its energy into flowering and will die once it has flowered in the summer.

### Burdock and dandelion root decoction

Simmer about an ounce each of fresh chopped **burdock and dandelion root** in 3 cups of **water** for 20 minutes. Strain and divide into three or four doses to drink during the day, hot or cold. If you want to sweeten it, add a tablespoonful of dried liquorice root before boiling.

### Burdock and dandelion toffee

Dig several roots of **burdock and dandelion**, in spring or fall. Strip the root bark off, and clean and chop up the inner part. Weigh out 3 to 4 ounces of each. Load into a saucepan and cover with **a pint of water**. Bring to a boil and simmer for 20 minutes. Allow to cool.

Simmer again until the roots are tasteless (i.e., have surrendered their content to the liquid). This reduces the mixture by about half. Strain and add **1 tablespoon butter and 12 tablespoons of sugar**. Boil for 5 minutes then simmer for 20 minutes more. It will become toffee-like. Test the toffee by pouring a drip of it onto a cold plate, as you would in testing jam: when it crinkles into soft threads, it is ready. Pour it into a buttered shallow tin. Before it sets totally, mark out squares and save the toffee slab in greaseproof paper; or stretch it out by hand into taffee: this is pale and pliable, ideal for balls, plaits, etc.

**Burdock leaf poultice**
- bruises
- boils
- acne
- rheumatism
- arthritis
- gout

**Burdock & dandelion root decoction**
- acne
- eczema
- boils
- psoriasis
- detoxing

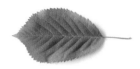

# Cherry *Prunus avium, P. serotina*

**Rosaceae**
**Rose family**

**Description:** Tall trees with smooth, shiny and red–brown bark, peeling horizontally; bearing soft white flowers in spring; mazzards have small red or yellow cherries while black cherries have dark purple cherries.

**Habitat:** Edges of woods and fields, backyards.

**Distribution:** Wild sweet cherries are native to Europe and naturalized in North America. North American wild cherry or black cherry is naturalized in Europe.

**Related species:** The sour or dwarf cherry (*P. cerasus*) yields sour Morello cherries. It is native to Europe but naturalized in North America. Like sweet cherry, it is often cultivated. Chokecherry (*P. virginiana*) bark can be used like black cherry, but the fruit needs to be cooked and sweetened to be palatable.

**Parts used:** Fruit and fruit stalks gathered in summer, bark harvested in fall.

Wild sweet cherries, also known as gaskins, geans, mazzards, and merrys, are not only delicious to eat but also good for your gout or arthritis. The fruit stalks and inner bark of sweet and black cherries have medicinal virtues too, for treating dry coughs, sore throats, and bronchitis. It is a bonus that children seem to love cherry tea or syrup, leaving their parents to drink up the home-made cherry brandy .

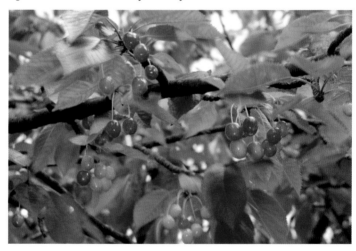

We all know and enjoy cherry blossom in spring and the cherry harvest later in the year, but this is a tree whose bark is as valuable as its flowers, fruit, and wood.

The official *British Herbal Pharmacopoeia* lists the powdered bark of the American black cherry (*P. serotina*) as an anti-tussive, i.e., anti-cough, remedy, but we have found wild sweet cherry bark to be very similar in use.

Long used as a country recipe, a decoction or syrup of the inner bark of wild cherry, alone or with elderberry (as in our recipe), plums, or sloes, is a tasty and safe drink for sore throats and bronchitis that children find palatable. Its special affinity is for dry and irritating coughs. The stalks of sweet cherries also have a traditional use as a decoction for coughs, with similar effects to the bark. The fruit can be added for flavor.

The fruit has a reputation as a gout treatment, but you would need to eat quite a lot of cherries to lower the high levels of uric acid implicated. Cherries work well as a gentle laxative, but anyone who has gorged on fresh cherries will have discovered that eating too many can cause diarrhea.

Cherries contain anthocyanins, which are potent antioxidants, as well as vitamins A, B, and C. They are cleansing and nourishing, and help to "build the blood" in cases of weakness and anemia. Eating cherries helps with colds and recovery from illness, and they taste so good you hardly need an excuse to eat them.

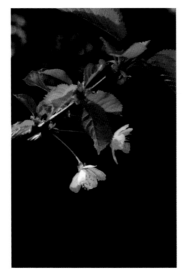

*The cherry tree is the only fruit tree I know where people hold the bark in as high esteem as the fruit.*
*– Brill & Dean (1994)*

*A tree of virtuous blossom, virtuous timber, and rather less virtuous fruit, except for the purposes of cherry brandy.*
*– Grigson (1958)*

**Fresh cherry fruit**
- anemia
- constipation
- gout
- arthritis

**Cherry bark and elderberry syrup**
- coughs
- sore throats
- bronchitis

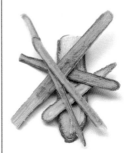

### Cherry brandy
Loosely fill a preserving jar with **cherries**. If they are sour, sprinkle with a little **muscovado sugar**, then top up the jar with **brandy**. Latch the lid down tightly and shake the jar well. Turn it upside down every few days to keep the sugar from settling at the bottom. After three months, strain and bottle. Enjoy at your leisure.

### Cherry bark and elderberry cough syrup
Cut thin strips of **bark** from cherry branches in the autumn when the leaves are falling. One way to do this is to prune off a few small branches, then use a sharp knife to cut off all the bark. It is the greenish-white inner bark that is medicinal. Dry the bark in the shade.

Fill a small jar with the **dried bark** and top it up with **vodka**. Leave in a cool dark place for a month, shaking the jar occasionally, then strain. This is a cherry bark tincture.

To make the cough syrup, combine 1 part **cherry bark tincture** with 2 parts **elderberry glycerite** (recipe, page 63).

**Dose:** 1 teaspoonful three or four times a day. Halve this for children.

Cherry     25

# Chickweed *Stellaria media*

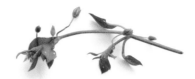

**This is the best-known herbal remedy for itchy skin and hot skin inflammations of various types. Chickweed is a soothing, nutritious, and cooling herb, with a reputation for clearing stubborn, long-lasting bodily conditions.**

**It has special affinities for the eyes, lungs, and chest, and can be eaten as a food. As you'll see, it is far more than chickenfeed!**

**Caryophyllaceae
Pink family**

**Description:** A floppy, sprawling annual plant with soft green leaves and tiny star-like white flowers.

**Habitat:** Gardens, hedgebanks, and waste ground.

**Distribution:** Native to Europe and Asia but now found as a weed worldwide.

**Related species:** There are over a hundred species in the genus.

**Parts used:** Above-ground parts, gathered whenever vibrant and green.

Chickweed has a number of less familar old names, such as chick wittles, clucken wort, and chickeny weed, which confirm it is as a fowl favorite. This fact can be attested worldwide: for example, Julie's grandmother in Australia had chickens that loved their chickweed. Matthew's mother in Cambridgeshire can vouch for the relish with which her caged canaries used to nibble fresh chickweed flowers and seeds. Not surprisingly, it is also called bird seed.

But why should birds have all the fun? Chickweed is an excellent salad plant for humans, especially in late winter and early spring, when there's little else green and fresh available for foraging.

It tastes as though it is full of chlorophyll, has an earthy, slightly salty tang, and is easily gathered. Its high vitamin A and C levels, saponins, and plentiful minerals, including iron, copper, magnesium, and calcium, make it one of the best spring tonics.

Chickweed has long been eaten fresh this way by country people and it was once sold in the streets of London. Chickweed is tender and juicy, and has been called the tenderest of wild greens.

We often harvest it fresh for salad. Chickweed on its own is perhaps an acquired taste, but it is bland and goes well in a mixed salad. The tastiest way we have found to eat it is to make it into a pesto with pine nuts, which is surprisingly good (see recipe).

Chickweed is available almost all year round, except in midsummer when it becomes fibrous and in midwinter when it disappears. It is one of the most genteel of weeds, easily pulled up and never rambunctious. Its presence signals fertile soil and it helps keep the soil moist. And once you find how good it is, you'll never seem to have enough of it!

One help in identifying chickweed among its *Stellaria* cousins

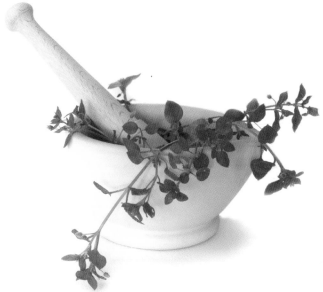

*In late winter, it's a blessing for victims of F.W.S. (Forager's Withdrawal Syndrome) who crave a wild salad.*
– Brill & Dean (1994)

*Think of chickweed as being as soft as slippery elm, as soothing as marshmallow, and as protective and strengthening as comfrey root.*
– Weed (1989)

is its very commonness, virtually around the world. Chickweed is a very floppy plant and has smooth light green leaves, with a single line of white hairs up the side of the stem. In any event, other members of its clan have similar herbal attributes, such as lots of vitamins A and C and steroidal saponins, and can be used safely, if somewhat less effectively.

## Use chickweed for...

Chickweed makes a good broth or tea for children and convalescents and can be taken in quantity. One American herbalist writes with gusto of taking "quarts of chickweed a day."

Herbally, the best-known external use for chickweed is to soothe itches, bites, stings, inflammations, burns, swellings, sunburn, bruises, splinters, and sore eyes. It makes a good and readily found first-aid or emergency remedy – pull up a handful and place directly onto the affected part. If you have a little more time, crush some chickweed with a mortar and pestle and bandage the paste against the wound or bite as a poultice. This is very cooling and soothing for sunburn.

Chickweed has the particular reputation of resolving skin problems where some form of heat is involved and where other herbs or creams have failed, especially when a cooling, drawing action is needed.

It is also known for clearing up long-standing or "indolent" damage, such as eczema, rheumatic joints, and varicose veins.

*This small herb, often classed as a troublesome weed, is one of the supreme healers of the herbal kingdom, and has given me wonderful results.*
– Levy (1966)

[The *Stellaria* species are an] ... *interesting group of plants that have rather fallen into disuse. The notable exception is chickweed without which a herbal dispensary is incomplete.*
– Barker (2001)

It is also safe for delicate organs that need cooling and soothing. One special affinity it has is for eye inflammations of most sorts, including itchiness from a contact lens. Dioscorides, the Greek scientist, described a chickweed recipe nearly two thousand years ago: he added crushed chickweed to corn meal to produce a paste that was poulticed onto the affected eye.

We mentioned before that chickweed contains saponins. Saponin means "soap-like." If you take a handful of the plant and rub it in your hands with a little water, you may not actually get a lather, but you'll feel the soapiness and it'll leave your hands feeling lovely and soft, if smelling a little of chickweed.

Saponins work at a cellular level to increase absorption and permeability. What this means is that inflamed organ membranes, as in the liver, kidneys, and lungs, are helped by saponins to absorb healing nutrients, as well as allowing their wastes and blockages to be more easily removed. Add to this the cooling qualities of chickweed, and you have a wonderful, subtle herbal cleanser and restorer at work, far beyond the familiar and dismissive uses for "itchiness."

Chickweed works well internally on hot inflammatory problems like gastritis, colitis, congested chest, blocked kidneys and gallbladder, and piles. It has an affinity for the lungs, for sore throats, bronchitis,

asthma, irritable dry cough, and other respiratory conditions.

Another quality you may have encountered is chickweed's reputed value as a slimming aid. Chickweed water or tea is an old wives' remedy for the overweight, and dried chickweed is indeed added to some proprietary slimming preparations.

What do herbalists say? Some believe it does work, as the saponins help to dissolve body fat; others note it stimulates urination, so will assist in shedding body moisture, which would contribute to weight loss. As with many treatments, what works for one person may not be effective for everyone.

Chickweed has a valuable toning action for the body's internal organs. In American herbalist Susun

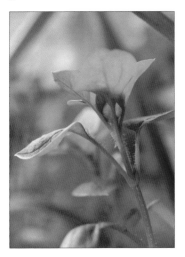

Weed's words, it "sponges up the spills" and "tidies up the rips." She refers to its "deep mending skills," and to its ability to relieve, clear, protect, and nourish.

Chickweed can also be made into a flower essence, which is used to help release the past and focus in the present moment. If you want to make a chickweed essence, follow the instructions on page 154.

Whether as a salad, tea or tincture, essence or vinegar, chickweed is effective, available, free, and safe.

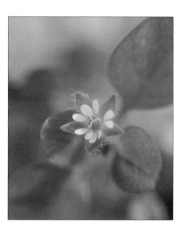

**Chickweed bath**
- itchy skin
- shingles
- rheumatism
- rashes

**Chickweed bath vinegar**
- itchy skin
- shingles
- rheumatism
- rashes

## Chickweed pesto

Pick a few handfuls of **chickweed**, removing any brown bits and roots. Break off the larger stems, as they have a very strong stretchy fiber at their core and are surprisingly stringy for such a floppy plant. Put the rest in a blender with a handful of **pine nuts**, a couple of cloves of **garlic**, and enough **olive oil** to make it blendable. Blend until it is as smooth as you like it, then serve fresh on pasta with some **grated pecorino or parmesan cheese**. It can also be eaten with rice or other grains, or used as a sauce for vegetables.

## Chickweed bath

For itchy skin, especially if this is over a large area of your body, try adding chickweed to a bath. Put a few handfuls of **fresh chickweed** in a sock or tie in a square of muslin, and use a piece of string to hang this under the hot tap so that the water flows through it as you run your bath. Oatmeal can also be mixed with the chickweed for additional soothing. Once the bath is run, gently squeeze the sock or bag to release more of the contents.

Alternatively, make a strong infusion of chickweed, strain, and add to the bath water.

## Chickweed bath vinegar

Pick **chickweed** and put it in a blender, adding enough **cider vinegar** to blend. Strain and bottle. Your vinegar will start out a light lime green and change after a day or two to a lovely golden color. Add a couple of tablespoons to bath water. This recipe combines chickweed's effectiveness at relieving itchy skin with vinegar's acidity, which helps restore the natural protective acid balance of the skin. It is particularly good if you live in a hard-water area.

Chickweed vinegar can also be used in salad dressings.

# Cleavers *Galium aparine*

**Also known as goose grass, clivers, and sticky-willy, this common roadside plant clambers all over hedges and other plants in a green mass in high summer. It sends up bright green shoots from January onward, being one of the first plants to sprout.**

**Cleavers is a wonderfully gentle lymphatic cleanser and a fantastic spring tonic, helping clean up our system after winter. It soothes irritated membranes of the urinary tract and promotes urine flow, and is useful for many mouth and throat problems.**

**Rubiaceae
Bedstraw family**

**Description:** A clambering annual covered in small hooks that help it "cleave" to anything it touches. Can be several yards high. Leaves are in whorls; small white flowers are followed by pairs of small ball-like fruit.

**Habitat:** Hedgerows, farmland, stream banks, and gardens.

**Distribution:** Native to Eurasia and North America; widespread but introduced in the southern hemisphere.

**Related species:** The genus *Galium* also includes the bedstraws. Lady's bedstraw (*G. verum*) and hedge bedstraw (*G. mollugo*) can be used interchangeably with cleavers as medicinal herbs.

**Parts used:** Aboveground parts, gathered in handfuls from early spring until the plants flower in the summer.

Cleavers is the earliest of the traditional spring tonic herbs to sprout, appearing even before the end of the year in sheltered spots under hedges. By February it is making dense mats of intensely green whorled leaves. This is the time to harvest it to eat in salads, before it becomes tough and hairy. Pick the shoots and chop them finely. Nicholas Culpeper (1653) nicely summarizes the traditional view:

*It is a good remedy in the Spring, eaten (being first chopped small, and boiled well) in water-gruel, to cleanse the blood, and strengthen the liver, thereby to keep the body in health, and fitting it for that change of season that is coming.*

By summer, cleavers romps all over the place, and its tiny white four-petaled flowers appear. At this stage, it will stick to anything, sometimes growing above head height. It can be used to make a quick makeshift collecting basket

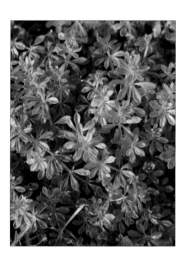

by twining it around on itself. As John Parkinson (1640) noted:

*the herbe serveth well the Country people in stead of a strainer, to cleare their milke from strawes, haires, or any other thing that falleth into it.*

To understand how cleavers works in the body, you need to know a little about the lymphatic system. When our arteries carry oxygenated blood out to the far reaches of the body, the blood vessels branch smaller and smaller until only one red blood cell at a time can pass through.

These tiny blood vessels are the capillaries. Here, the red blood cells give up their oxygen and nutrients to the clear liquid around them, which then crosses the capillary walls into the cells.

The cells take the oxygen and nutrients, and in return give up their metabolic waste products to the fluid. This fluid doesn't go back into the blood vessels, but is collected by the lymphatic vessels, which are like a white bloodstream flowing back through the body toward the heart in parallel with the veins.

White blood cells in the lymphatic fluid start cleaning it up, and it passes through lymph nodes where the process continues. When it is all clean, the fluid rejoins the bloodstream at the point where the large vein enters the heart. Here it is pumped out to the lungs and the cycle begins again. If the lymph is clean and flowing well, the body will be healthy.

### Use cleavers for...
Herbally, cleavers promotes the lymphatic flow and helps rid the lymphatic system of metabolic waste. In effect, it is like a pipe cleaner for the body's lymph ves-

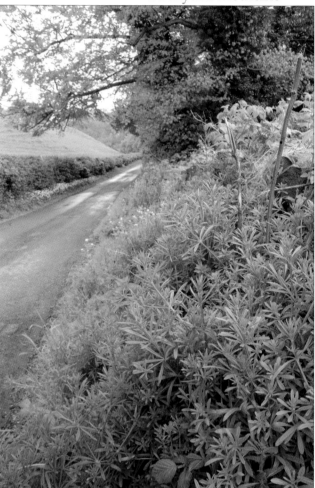

A spring tonic in the raw: cleavers in foreground, ramsons flowering across the road on left. In County Durham, northern England

sels. This makes it a good remedy for swollen glands, adenoid problems, tonsillitis, and earache. Again because of its effect on the lymph, cleavers enjoys a strong reputation for helping to shrink tumors, both benign and cancerous, and for removing nodular growths on the skin.

*It is wonderful how strong and healthy you will become* [on taking cleavers juice mixed with spring water]
– The Physicians of Myddfai (13th century)

Austrian herbalist Maria Treben (1980) favored cleavers tea as a drink and gargle to treat cancers of the tongue and throat. It is good too for other problems of the tongue, throat, and neck, and is used by herbalists for goitre, other thyroid issues, and swollen glands.

Because it promotes the flow of urine, and is cooling and soothing, cleavers is used to reduce heat and irritation of the urinary tract. It relieves the scalding pain on urination associated with cystitis, and is a remedy for chronic recurrent bouts of urethritis, for kidney inflammation, irritable bladder, and prostatitis.

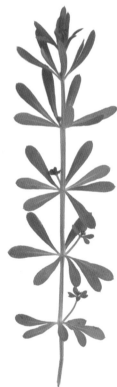

It is also effective in clearing grit, gravel or calcium deposits in the urinary tract. As a bonus, because cleavers is so good at cleaning the body internally, it also helps clear and nourish the skin.

Cleavers combines well with other familiar "weeds" – curly dock, nettle, dandelion, and burdock – as in our "garden weed tincture" recipe. This tincture is an effective cleansing tonic for the whole body.

Cleavers loses some of its effectiveness when dried, and works best fresh. Picking your own in the spring and using it daily while in season is a great way to give yourself a gentle annual spring-cleanse. Try chopping a little young cleavers to mix in with salads or add to soups. The juice can be blended with fruit smoothies.

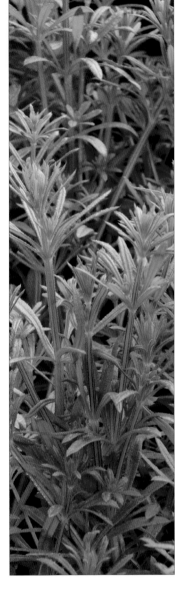

### Cleavers poultice

The fresh, bruised plant is an excellent poultice for nettle rash, sores, blisters, burns, or any hot inflammation of the skin. Just pick a handful of cleavers, crush it with a mortar and pestle, and apply to the skin.

### Cleavers juice

Taking the fresh juice is the best way to use cleavers from early spring until summer. If you don't have a juicer, don't worry – just chop up a handful of fresh cleavers, put it in a jelly bag, and squeeze out the juice.
**Dose:** Take 1 teaspoonful two or three times a day.

### Cleavers succus

If you want to preserve your cleavers juice for use in the autumn and winter, the best way is to mix it with glycerine or honey to make a simple preparation called a succus. This is done as follows:

Measure your fresh **cleavers juice**, and add an equal amount of **vegetable glycerine** or **runny honey**. Mix well, then bottle and label. It tastes just like the smell of fresh-mown grass.

**Dose:** Take 1 to 2 teaspoonfuls two or three times a day.

### Cleavers ointment

Stir the **fresh juice** into **anhydrous lanolin** until it is soft and a pale green color. Use a fork for this. It's hard work at first, but gets easier as the lanolin starts to absorb the juice. This is a particularly good application for dry, cracked, or chapped skin.

### Garden weed tincture

Here's a great way to turn a morning's weeding into something really useful – a whole-body tonic to improve your health generally.
Weed out and wash:
**Cleavers** – best collected before they set seed
**Dandelion plants** – root, leaves, and all
**Nettle tops** (before they flower) and **nettle root**
**Curled dock roots**
**Burdock roots**
Chop the herbs and put them in a large, wide-mouthed jar, packing them in fairly tightly. Pour on enough **vodka** to cover them, and leave for a month, shaking occasionally. Strain off. If you have a fruit press, use it to get the maximum liquid out of the roots; otherwise just use muscle power to squeeze it out using a jelly bag. Bottle and label.

**Dose:** 1 teaspoonful twice a day.

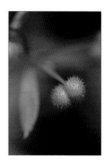

**Cleavers in salads**
• spring tonic

**Cleavers poultice**
• sunburn
• burns
• psoriasis
• open sores
• blisters
• nettle rash

**Cleavers juice**
• swollen glands
• fluid retention
• tonsillitis
• breast cysts
• bladder irritation
• burning urine

**Cleavers succus**
• swollen glands
• fluid retention
• tonsillitis
• breast cysts
• bladder irritation
• burning urine

**Cleavers ointment**
• dry chapped skin
• chapped lips
• burns

**Garden weed tincture**
• skin problems
• weak digestion
• anemia
• low energy

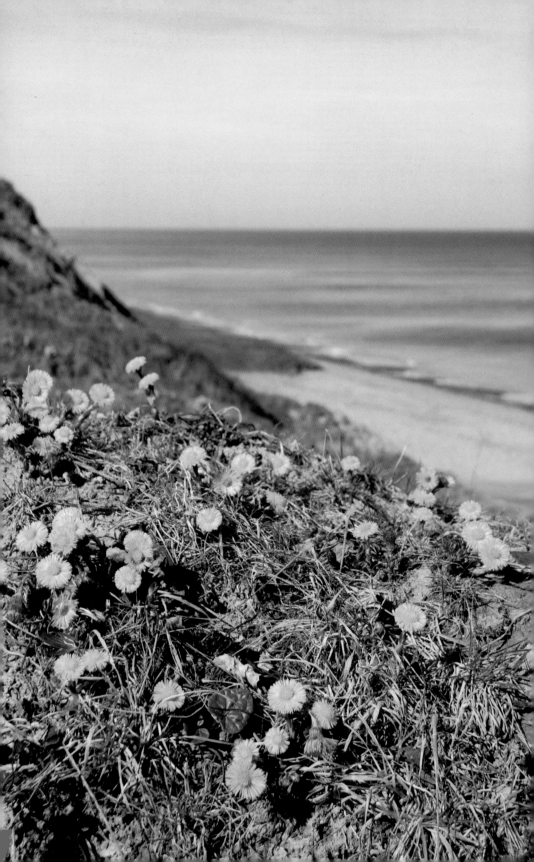

# Coltsfoot *Tussilago farfara*

**Asteraceae
(Compositae)
Daisy family**

**Coltsfoot is one of the earliest plants of the herbalist's year, and its leaves and flowers make an effective cough remedy.**

**Description:** A perennial herb that flowers in late winter/early spring before the heart-shaped polygonal leaves appear.

Coltsfoot is found in profusion locally on roadsides, slopes, and stream banks and is one of the first plants to appear in early spring. It yields flowers before leaves, a fact reflected in the old name "son before the father." Coltsfoot is unmistakable when in flower, but its large, roughly heart-shaped leaves can be confused with the related butterbur in summer, so be sure you have the right plant.

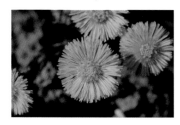

**Habitat:** Stream banks, roadsides, paths, cliffs, woodland, and waste ground.

**Distribution:** Native to Europe and northern Asia; naturalized in North America. Note the prohibitions on its use in certain East and West Coast US states.

Both flowers and leaves are used medicinally, and the Latin names tell us so. *Tussilago* is from the Latin *tussis* for cough, and *farfara* or flour refers to the whitish, cottony down on the underside of the leaves. Before commercial matches were available, this down was collected and dipped into a solution of saltpeter for use in tinder-boxes.

**Related species:** In summer, coltsfoot leaves can be mistaken for butterbur (*Petasites hybridus*) and winter heliotrope (*P. fragrans*), which should not be used.

**Parts used:** Flowers in early spring, leaves gathered in summer.

It is the leaves that give coltsfoot its name. As well as colts or foals, they have also been named for the hooves of bulls, pigs, and even asses. The flowers are succeeded by dandelion-like clocks made up of tiny white seed parachutes.

A bright sunny March morning saw us by the sea in north-eastern Norfolk (UK), where the clay cliffs were covered in maritime mini-meadows of sunny yellow. Here coltsfoot is a dominant plant, a colonizer and stabilizer of a crumbling, eroding coastline. An inspiring sight to eyes bereft of color and sunlight through a long winter! The bees and hover flies were gorging on the sweet nectar, and seeing these swathes of sunshine you could finally believe spring was really back again.

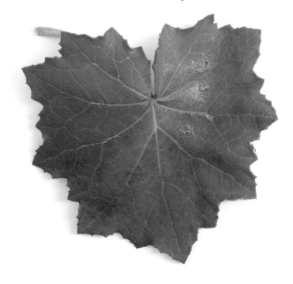

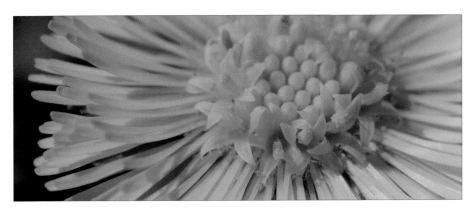

### Use coltsfoot for ...

Coltsfoot has long been used for all kinds of cough and upper respiratory tract complaints. The flowers and leaves yield a sweetish, aniseedish tea, taken separately or together, fresh or dried. Some herbalists advise straining the tea to remove the leaf hairs, which can be an irritant.

It was an interesting coincidence for us that at the time we photographed the coltsfoot meadows Julie was suffering a hacking cough, so we gathered some flowers to make tea, which was just what she needed. It is very soothing, calming a cough almost at once. It helps moisten a dry irritating cough and loosen phlegm.

Coltsfoot leaves have also been used as a smoking tobacco since classical Greek and Roman times (respectively, Dioscorides and Pliny write about it), and have earned the name "British tobacco." You can use the dried leaves to roll your own or smoke them in a pipe – proving that you can sometimes smoke to alleviate a cough!

Coltsfoot "rock" is an old-fashioned and pleasant-tasting commercially available confection. This is a good way to persuade children to take a cough remedy. And coltsfoot was usually the first wild flower available to make a light wine, appearing even before cowslip.

Coltsfoot has been found to contain pyrrolizidine alkaloids, as does comfrey. Not all these alkaloids are toxic, however, and coltsfoot's small amounts do not appear to be harmful at low doses. As cough remedies are not normally taken long-term anyway, there is little chance of coltsfoot causing any problems. To be safe, we suggest taking it for no more than six weeks in total in a year.

Coltsfoot combines well with mullein, especially for dry coughs, and is good as a tea with fennel.

*This is the cough remedy* par excellence *and is safe and effective for children providing that it is taken only for temporary symptomatic use.*
*– Barker (2001)*

### Coltsfoot and fennel tea

While coltsfoot can be used on its own as a tea, it is tastier and even more soothing when combined with fennel. You can use it fresh or dried to make this tea. To dry coltsfoot, spread the flowers or leaves on a screen or a tray and put it in a warm cupboard until they are crisp. Store in brown paper bags, or in a jar in a cool dark cupboard.

Put **four or five coltsfoot flowers or a couple of leaves** in a teapot with a **heaped teaspoonful of fennel seed**. Pour boiling water over them and brew for 10 minutes, then strain and drink hot.

**Dose:** Drink a cupful three times a day. It is wonderfully soothing for coughs and bronchial inflammation.

### Coltsfoot and honey poultice

Mix the **chopped leaves** with enough **honey** to make a paste, and apply to boils and sores that won't heal. Place a piece of gauze over the poultice, and bandage in place. Change for a fresh poultice every day until healed.

**Coltsfoot tea**
• coughs
• bronchitis
• throat irritation
• mild asthma

**Coltsfoot poultice**
• boils
• sores
• ulcers

**Cautions**
In view of its pyrrolizidine alkaloid content, coltsfoot should not be used for more than six weeks a year in total. Do not use if pregnant or breastfeeding, or give to young children.

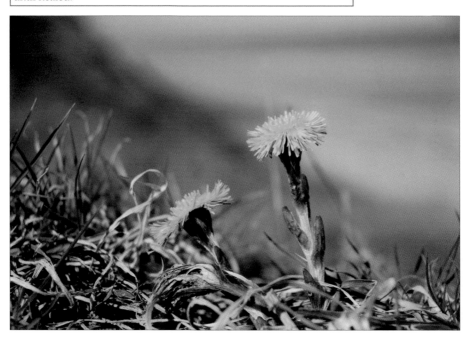

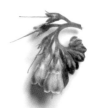

**Boraginaceae
Borage family**

**Description:** A lush, hairy, fast-growing plant with yellowish-cream or dull purple flowers, and a winged stem.

**Habitat:** Moist, marshy places.

**Distribution:** Native through Europe to Siberia. Introduced to North America and other temperate regions.

**Related species:** There are a number of species, often found as garden escapes. They can all be used externally, but only *Symphytum officinale* should be taken internally. Russian comfrey (*S.* x *uplandicum*) prefers drier ground, and is a hybrid between common comfrey (*S. officinale*) and rough or prickly comfrey (*S. asperum*). Tuberous comfrey (*S. tuberosum*) has pale yellowish-cream flowers. Because comfreys hybridize, it can be difficult to tell them apart.

**Parts used:** Leaves, root.

# Comfrey *Symphytum officinale*

**Comfrey's old name of knitbone refers to its strong healing action for broken bones. It will also knit flesh together, speeding the healing of wounds. Applied as a poultice or ointment, it can be used to treat bruises, dislocations, and sprains. Despite much controversy, comfrey is safe if correct guidelines are followed.**

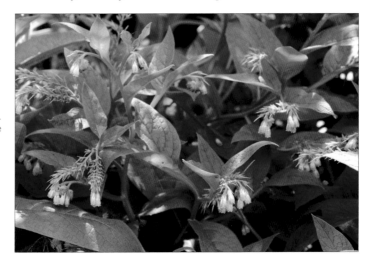

Comfrey has a long history of use for its healing and anti-inflammatory effects on bone fractures, arthritis, inflamed joints, cuts, wounds, and other injuries.

This herb had such a reputation for repairing tissue that it was said that less virtuous brides would bathe in comfrey before their wedding day to restore their virginity!

Both comfrey's scientific and common names refer to its healing qualities. *Symphytum* is from the Greek *symphyo*, make grow together, and *phyton*, plant; "comfrey" is said to be from the Roman word *conferre*, join together.

In addition to its medicinal benefits, comfrey is often grown as a fodder plant for animals, as a fertilizer and to add to compost. The most commonly grown comfrey for these purposes is Bocking 14, a sterile clone of Russian comfrey (*S.* x *uplandicum*).

### Use comfrey for ...

In the past, comfrey was widely used for healing ulceration in the digestive tract, as it is mucilaginous and soothing as well as healing. It was also used for bronchitis and other chest complaints, to soothe the irritation and promote expectoration of mucus.

Today, other herbs tend to be preferred for these conditions, owing to the possible dangers of the pyrrolizidine alkaloids contained in comfrey – see box on page 40. Comfrey nonetheless remains valuable as one of the best herbs for healing broken bones, snapped tendons, sprains, strains, and bruises.

Once a bone has been set by a qualified person, apply a fresh comfrey poultice. If the fracture is in plaster, take the comfrey up to the edges of the plaster. In addition, use homeopathic comfrey (Symphytum 6x) internally as directed by a homeopath, or – as long as you are not pregnant or breastfeeding – you can drink a couple of cups of comfrey leaf tea a day until the bone heals. Use a leaf or half a large leaf per cup of tea, infusing for 5 minutes.

Comfrey can also be applied to varicose veins, as a poultice. For wounds and ulcers that are open, place mashed comfrey on the skin around the affected part. Comfrey can help heal old wounds such as surgical scars, being applied as a fresh poultice or using the infused

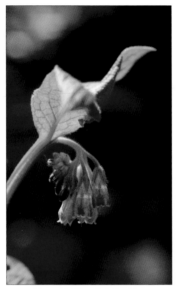

oil or ointment. It is also effective on bruises and other injuries to the muscles, ligaments and tendons.

Comfrey's powerful healing effects are partly explained by its allantoin content. This chemical stimulates cell proliferation, which speeds up the healing process, and is also an anti-inflammatory that supports the immune system.

Comfrey is so good at "knitting" that it must not be used on broken bones until they have been set, or it will start bonding them together in the wrong position. Likewise, do not apply it on deep wounds, which can close at the top before the deep part has healed underneath. St John's wort is better for deep puncture wounds.

*Comfery roots scrapd & boyle in milk is good to eat at night going to bed for a strayn or crik in the back; and boyld in ale to the thickness of a poultice [is] good to aply to a strayn.*
*– handwritten recipe from Norfolk, eighteenth century*

*It does not seem to matter much which part of the body is broken, either internally or externally; comfrey will heal it quickly.*
*– Dr Shook (quoted by Dr Christopher, 1976)*

**Cautions:** Do not use comfrey root internally, and do not take comfrey leaf for longer than six weeks at a time. Do not use internally if pregnant or breastfeeding, or give to young children. The FDA recommends that comfrey is not used internally at all.

**Mistaken identities:** Foxglove (*Digitalis purpurea*) leaves can easily be confused with comfrey before the plants flower.

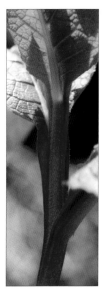

Common comfrey's leaves run down the stem to the joint below, giving the stem a winged appearance

**Common comfrey** is the commonest comfrey in wetter habitats, but the flower color is very variable, ranging from creamy white through pink to dull purple. The leaves run down onto the stem, with the upper leaves extending right down to the next set of leaves, giving the stem a winged appearance (see photo left).

**Russian comfrey** is the most common comfrey in drier places. Its flowers are bright blue or purple, and the upper stem leaves don't run down the stem, or do so only slightly. **Rough comfrey**, its other parent plant, has bluish flowers and the upper stem leaves have short stalks and never run down the stem.

### Comfrey and the pyrrolizidine alkaloid controversy

Comfrey has come into disrepute in recent years because it contains pyrrolizidine alkaloids. This is a large group of chemicals, some of which are toxic to the liver and can cause hepatic veno-occlusive disease. Poisoning has been reported in people eating other plants with high levels of these alkaloids, and there are a few reported cases of liver damage that appear to be based on the use of comfrey root.

Some herbalists argue that comfrey has been used traditionally and safely for hundreds of years without any problems, but the other side of the argument is that damage could occur gradually over time and not be attributed to the herb.

Another factor is the fact that Russian comfrey has been promoted for its benefits as a fertilizer and in making compost, especially for organic gardeners. It is wonderful for this purpose, but the problem from a medicinal point of view is that this is now the comfrey that most people have growing in their gardens.

Its levels of pyrrolizidine alkaloids are much higher than those of common comfrey, the "official" species of herbalism. Russian comfrey is a hybrid between common comfrey and rough or prickly comfrey. Russian comfrey and prickly comfrey contain echimidine, the most toxic of the alkaloids, and are best limited to external use. The species hybridize readily and can be difficult to tell apart, but see above for guidelines. Growing conditions probably also have an effect on alkaloid levels, making the issue more complex.

It is better to err on the side of caution rather than risk any problems, so it is recommended that no comfrey root be used internally (it contains higher levels of alkaloids than the leaves). External use on unbroken skin is considered safe.

Common comfrey leaf can certainly be safely taken internally for short periods. Six weeks at a time is long enough to heal a broken bone.

Bisset and Wichtl (2001) say that a high level of consumption of the leaves "as a salad is five or six leaves a day," which would be within the toxic range. Using a couple of leaves a day to make tea should be fine for short-term use, and herbalist Susun Weed says she has been drinking more than a quart a week for 20 years with no ill effects.

Do not take comfrey internally during pregnancy, while breastfeeding or if you have liver disease.

### Fresh comfrey poultice

Dig up **comfrey roots** and scrub them well. Cut them into shorter lengths and put them in a blender with an equal amount of **fresh comfrey leaf**. Add just enough water to make it blendable, and blend until you have a gooey mess. Spread this onto a piece of gauze and apply to the body part affected, covering with a piece of muslin or cling-film. The gauze makes the poultice easier to remove. Replace poultice daily until healed.

The leaves can also be used on their own as a poultice, but the hairs on them can irritate the skin. To avoid this, blend the leaves with a little water or pound them in a mortar and pestle, and then sandwich the leaf mush between two pieces of muslin before applying to the skin. The muslin will protect the skin from the irritating effects of the leaf hairs, and allow the juices to seep through.

### Infused comfrey oil

Pick **comfrey leaves** and let them dry in the shade; then crumble them up and put into a jar big enough to hold them. Pour in **extra virgin olive oil**, and stir well. Top up the jar with a little more oil, put the lid on and place in a sunny part of the garden or on a windowsill for two weeks. Strain off the oil and bottle it, or use it to make an ointment (below).

### Comfrey ointment

Put 10 fl oz of **infused comfrey oil** (above) in a small saucepan with 1 oz **beeswax**. The beeswax will melt faster if you grate it or slice it up. Warm up on low heat until the beeswax melts. Allow to cool slightly, then pour into jars and leave to set before putting the lids on and labeling.

**Comfrey poultice**
- broken bones
- sprains
- sports injuries
- bruises
- surgical scars

**Infused comfrey oil, ointment**
- arthritis
- rheumatism
- bursitis
- tendonitis
- phlebitis
- mastitis
- glandular swellings
- pulled muscles
- injured joints
- back injuries
- tendons
- ligaments

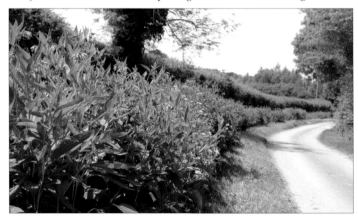

Russian comfrey (*S.* x *uplandicum*) growing along a country lane in Norfolk, England in July

# Couch grass *Elytrigia repens*, syn. *Elymus repens, Agropyron repens, Triticum repens*

**This invasive grass is both gardener's or farmer's foe and herbalist's friend. The couch grass rhizomes that gardeners hate possess soothing, diuretic, and antibiotic qualities that have long been valued for making a tea to treat urinary problems, including cystitis, kidney stones, and prostate enlargement.**

**Gramineae
Grass family**

**Description:** A grass, up to 3 feet tall, with a thin flowering spike, dark green pointed leaves, and untidy creeping rhizomes.

**Habitat:** Lawns and gardens, roadsides and fields.

**Distribution:** Widespread worldwide, in a large range of habitats. Common across North America. Declared an invasive weed in many US states.

**Related species:** Bermuda grass (*Cynodon dactylon*), common in warmer areas, is also sometimes known as couch grass, and is used medicinally.

**Parts used:** Rhizome.

Garden weeds often attract colorful names that leave little doubt about gardeners' opinions. Couch grass is no exception, its other common names including twitch, quick grass, quack grass, scutch grass, dog's grass, witch grass, and foul grass. It quickly spreads in most soils by vigorous white rhizomes (*repens* means creeping) just below the surface and forms a strong, dense root network that crowds out other plants.

Yet its herbal use goes back to classical times, and the love/hate relationship must also be as old. Culpeper, in 1653, puts it like this: "although a gardener be of another opinion, yet a physician holds half an acre of them [dog's grass or couch grass] to be worth five acres of Carrots twice told over."

The name "couch," according to the herbals, derives from an Anglo-Saxon word, *civice*, for vivacious and long-lasting. Perhaps the herbalists won naming rights here, and it's best to celebrate the vigor of the plant and hope this might transfer to us when we use it.

A successful colonist in garden and field, as are all of our familiar weeds, couch grass has an almost unstoppable capacity to spread. The pale runners or rhizomes give off side branches at intervals of only a few inches, and at each node the plant sends up a new shoot and drops a new web of fine roots. The leading runner is described by one writer as a lance that forces its way through any obstacle, including within your prized blooms. And if you leave the tiniest particle of the plant as you pull it or dig it up, it will invariably grow back.

Couch grass is sometimes confused with perennial rye grass (*Lolium perenne*), but this has a wavier flower stalk and alternating darkish green spikelets set close to the stalk. Couch grass has distinct, very flat pale green spikes set at an acute angle to the stem.

At least couch grass is valued in dryland Australia, being planted there to create durable golf courses, grass courts, and cricket squares. The binding quality of its rooting system has also been embraced in securing sand dunes, alongside specialist sand grasses.

And while gardeners in Britain may curse and burn their twitch, in mainland Europe it has often been used as a food for cows and horses, and sold as a tisane or tea for human use.

Mike Jones, a coffee plantation manager in Kenya for 26 years, now living in England, used to spend a month every year getting his workforce to dig out the couch grass by the deepest roots and burn it, or else it would climb to the top of the coffee bushes. When Julie sent him some couch grass, he said, "It comes as a bit of a surprise to learn we could have made ourselves a 'cup of tea' out of it."

What has so often been discarded should be more valued because it can ease a lot of suffering, and even prevent the need for surgery in some cases. A patient of Julie's, a keen gardener, said when prescribed couch grass, "But I've burned wheelbarrow loads of it!" He resolved to make better use of it in the future.

### Use couch grass for...
The same rhizomes that cause all the gardener's woes are dug up by herbalists, cleaned, dried, and cut into lengths of a few inches. Brewed as a tea, the resulting infusion is mild and pleasant to drink. It is an effective and long-proven remedy for cystitis, urethritis, and

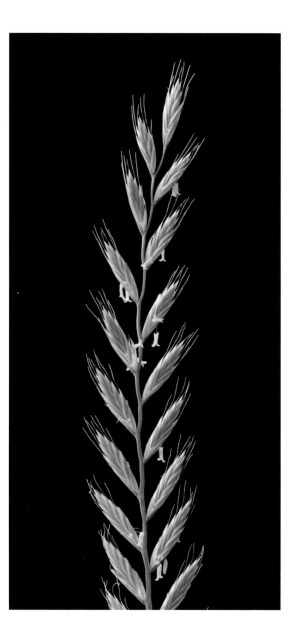

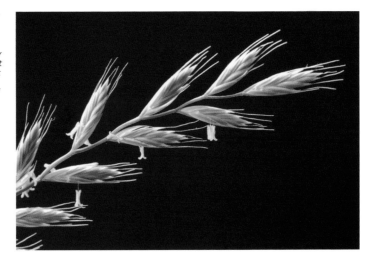

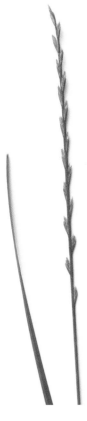

prostatitis, combining anti-microbial action with soothing and diuretic properties. In fact, it is almost a urinary formula all in one herb, as it also helps dissolve stones and gravel, as well as preventing them from building up.

John Parkinson, writing in 1640, said that couch grass (or Quich grasse, as he called it) not only dissolved stones in the bladder, but opened "obstructions of the liver and gall," indicating that it might help dissolve gallstones as well.

But it has wider modern uses too. Commission E, the expert panel that judges the safety of herbal medicines for the German government, has approved couch grass in the treatment of bronchitis and laryngitis as well as for bladder infections and kidney stones. It is also used together with other herbs for gout and rheumatism.

There are various other instances of couch grass being employed in European medicine for liver and gallbladder problems, including jaundice.

Dogs and cats will seek it out as a natural purgative (hence "dog's grass"). Horse owners add couch grass rhizomes to feed to improve their horses' coats.

Couch grass is untidy in habit, with dead brown leaves typically growing in a clump alongside the flowering spikes, as in the image opposite, but in supporting its claim on your attention, we invite you to take a look at the geometric beauty of the flowers in close-up (above and page 43).

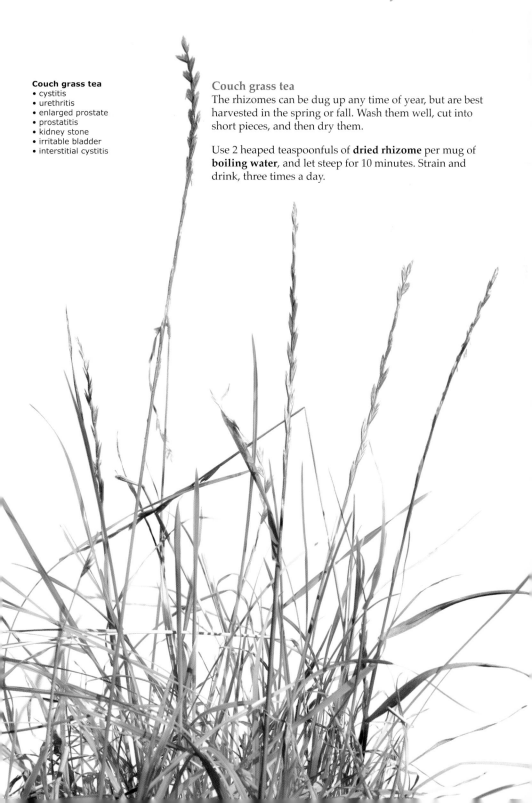

**Couch grass tea**
- cystitis
- urethritis
- enlarged prostate
- prostatitis
- kidney stone
- irritable bladder
- interstitial cystitis

Couch grass tea
The rhizomes can be dug up any time of year, but are best harvested in the spring or fall. Wash them well, cut into short pieces, and then dry them.

Use 2 heaped teaspoonfuls of **dried rhizome** per mug of **boiling water**, and let steep for 10 minutes. Strain and drink, three times a day.

# Curled dock, Yellow dock *Rumex crispus*

**Polygonaceae
Dock family**

**Description:** A perennial dock growing to a yard tall. Leaves are long and parallel-sided with wavy margins; tap roots have a brown outer covering and are yellow within.

**Habitat:** Grassland, disturbed ground, farmyards, roadsides, river banks, coastal shingle, and mud.

**Distribution:** Native to Europe and Africa, curled dock is one of the most widely distributed plants in North America and the world.

**Related species:** The other common species is common or broad-leaved dock (*R. obtusifolius*), with which yellow dock hybridizes. The root can be used interchangeably with curled dock – the thing to look for is a yellow root in either species, as that indicates the presence of the medicinal compounds.

**Parts used:** Root, dug up in fall; leaves.

Curled dock and broad-leaved dock are among the five official "injurious weeds" in Britain, but curled or yellow dock has long-recognized redeeming qualities as a detoxifying liver and bowel herb, a laxative, and a blood cleanser. The root is effective for many chronic toxic skin conditions, including acne and boils, eczema and sunburn, not forgetting the most famous use of dock leaves for relieving the burning caused by nettle stings.

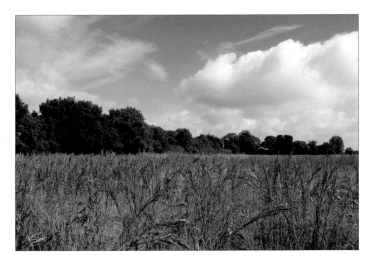

We have included dock in this book even though it is the root that is most used, as it is such a common weed across the world. Found in almost every field, garden, and lawn, it is likely you have some growing on your own plot that you can dig up for medicine.

Dock's tap roots are long, slender, and deep, going two feet down;

any stray piece left in the soil can sprout into a new plant. Each dock can produce 30,000 or more seeds a year, and these can lay dormant for up to fifty years. It is no wonder it is hard to eliminate. In addition, curled dock and common or broad-leaved dock hybridize freely. It is an almost unstoppable weed, yet one with redeeming medicinal benefits.

Dock's botanical success is official: both common British species are classed as injurious weeds in the Weeds Act 1959 (along with common ragwort, spear thistle, and creeping or field thistle). The Act stipulates that farmers should take steps to prevent the spread of these five weeds: a scene like the one opposite of a fallow field filled with curled dock in fall ought to be harder to find than it still is.

### Use curled dock for...

The one thing everybody knows about dock is that you rub its leaves on the skin when stung by nettle. This practice goes back centuries, being mentioned in the Anglo-Saxon leech-books and in Chaucer's *Troilus and Criseyde*, suggesting docks have always been freely available. Formerly, a chant was sung when applying the dock: in Ireland, it was "docken, docken, cure nettle"; in Cornwall, it was along the lines of "dock leaf, dock leaf, you go in; sting nettle, sting nettle, you come out."

It is a cooling and astringent treatment, especially the sizeable leaves of broad-leaved dock, although we prefer treating nettle rash by plantain leaves. Digging up a few dock roots, pulping them and applying as a poultice, and renewing this every few hours, is another old nettle standby, as is a root tea. In South Africa, Tswana women warm up dock leaves and apply them to swollen breasts during lactation; they also use the root pulp to treat piles.

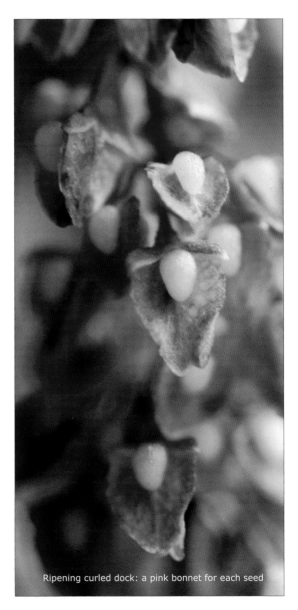

Ripening curled dock: a pink bonnet for each seed

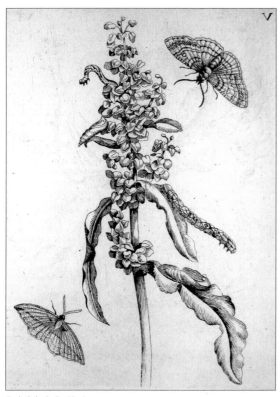

Curled dock, by Maria Merian (1717)

*Probably the most general practice in all of folk medicine, occurring throughout the British Isles, is rubbing a dock leaf on the skin to ease a sting.*
– Allen & Hatfield (2004)

The reputation of dock as a "blood cleanser" is also ancient, being known in Chinese medicine, Indian Ayurveda, and in classical Greece, whence comes dock's old family name "lapathum" or blood purifier. It was found that dock transmutes iron in the soil to organic iron in the plant (a real case of alchemy!); old herbalists would add iron filings to soil near dock to "enrich" it. This property makes dock effective for iron-deficiency anemia and for period problems, especially in younger women.

Dock also has a laxative effect in which it stimulates gut motions; indeed it was once used as a purgative. It is a good natural remedy for constipation, reflux, and acid stomach, and has been called a "superlative remedy" for enteritis, colitis, diarrhea, and dysentery.

Dock's twin qualities to cleanse and to lower heat make it an ideal liver detox treatment, including for jaundice and "liver stagnation," when the flow of bile is congested, and for disorders of the spleen and lymph. A healthy liver means a healthy skin, and dock works on both; the advice is to use small quantities over a long period.

One Anglo-Saxon recipe for reducing a groin swelling (attention, you sportsmen!) was to pulp dock leaves in grease, wrap in a cabbage leaf that had been warmed in hot ashes, and apply as a plaster. Culpeper (1653) suggested boiling roots in vinegar for bathing itches, scabs and "breaking out of the skin." Modern external uses have added chronic acne, boils, bites, cuts, sunburn, easing rheumatic aches, and soothing inflamed gums (using a powder of dried roots).

Dock root gives a gluten-free flour, once a famine food. The young leaves of curled dock cook as a tasty spring vegetable with a light lemony taste, and are good in nettle soup. Avoid too much raw dock, though, as it contains oxalic

## Harvesting dock

Dig up the roots in late summer or autumn. Large older plants are more likely to have a strong yellow color to their roots. Scrub them well, and cut off the tops.

## Curled dock tincture

Fill a jar with chopped-up **dock roots**. Pour **vodka** in until the roots are covered and put the lid on tightly. Keep in a cool dark place for a month, ideally shaking the jar every day or two.

Strain off, using a press or squeezing through a jelly bag. Bottle the liquid, remembering to label it. This tincture will keep for about five years in a cool dark place.

**Dose:** Half a teaspoonful once or twice daily as a cleansing tonic.

Take when the bowels are sluggish, for anemia and poor absorption of nutrients (if the edge of your tongue shows scalloping from your teeth), for skin problems, and any time you feel a bit slow and tired.

**Curled dock tincture**
- poor absorption
- anemia
- skin problems
- sluggish bowels
- liver congestion
- constipation

Curled dock root in cross-section, showing the yellow color

**An East Anglian cure for jaundice**
(collected by Elizabeth Hicks, late eighteenth century)

*Take 1 oz of red Doc. Seed dry, boil it in 3 pints of water till 1 pint is nearly wasted then strain it off and add 3 gill glasses of white Wine.*
*Dose take a gill glass 3 times a day when the stomach is the emptiest, this will be 4 days in taken, then stop 2 days and repeat the Medicine which will with the Blessing of God compleat the Cure be the Jaundice ever so bad.*

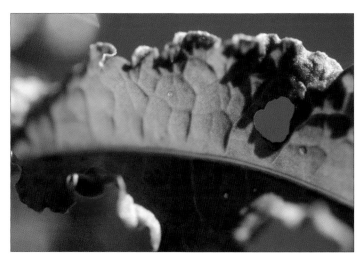

The wavy leaf edge (and typical snail hole) of curled dock

# Dandelion *Taraxacum officinale*

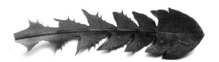

**Dandelion is a wonderful food as well as a beneficial medicine. It supports overall health by gently working to improve the functioning of the liver, gallbladder, and urinary and digestive systems. It is excellent for cleansing the skin.**

**Next time you spend an hour removing dandelions from your garden or lawn, turn them into medicine instead of throwing them out, and rejoice in the fact that they will always grow back!**

**Asteraceae (Compositae) Daisy family**

**Description:** A familiar weed of lawns, with bright yellow flowers, seed "clocks," a bitter white latex in the stem, and a long tap root.

**Habitat:** Lawns, fields, and roadside verges.

**Distribution:** Worldwide in temperate zones.

**Related species:** *Taraxacum officinale* is actually a group of several hundred plants. These are divided into nine sections and are very difficult to distinguish. The most common dandelions belong to the *Ruderalia* section. They are all safe medicinal plants. In Chinese medicine, *T. mongolicum* is used to clear heat and toxicity.

**Parts used:** Leaves, roots, flowers, and sap.

Dandelions: where to begin? They do so much! They were once much used in Britain as a spring tonic, and still are in Europe. In the US fresh dandelion leaves for salads was a three-million-dollar-a-year industry in 1999.

Dandelions have followed European settlers around the world, though it is probably native in China and most of Asia. Most people know them as lawn weeds, but we're prepared to upset the gardeners to say: consider the benefits of a lawn of brightly blooming dandelions. Can grass give you salad, tasty fritters, wine, a coffee substitute, tea, useful medicine and more besides?

This plant is almost indestructible: it is a perennial and, unusually, it is self-fertilizing; its deep tap roots make it hard to dig out, and any pieces left will regenerate. Its seeds soar miles on little parachutes, whether or not helped by children playing the "clock" game. It flowers almost all year long.

Any amount of mowing, herbicide, and flamethrowing fail to eradicate this sunny plant from the garden. Really, you'll be happier if you view dandelions as a culinary and medicinal gift, a superb "cut and come again" crop, rather than as an annoying weed!

An old companion of man, it has accumulated many names. Blowball and telltime refer to the seeds, priest's crown to the stem after the seeds have flown, and swine's snout to the unopened flower. And "dandelion" itself? The "teeth of the lion" (*dent de lion*) explanation, from the appearance of the saw-edged leaves or perhaps the tiny florets, is found in many languages. But there is also a case made for an older link to the sun.

In many cultures the lion has been the animal symbol of the sun since antiquity, as in the astrological sign Leo. Dandelions are yellow disks, like the sun, and open and close along with it. So, perhaps

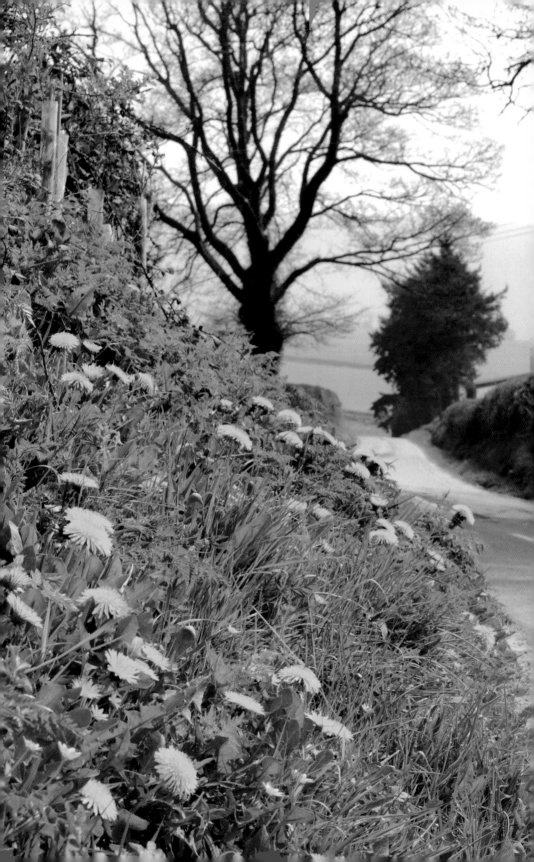

*It is very effectual for the obstructions of the liver, gall and spleen, and the distempers that arise therefrom, jaundice and the hypo-chondriacal passion. It wonderfully opens the urinary tract.*
– Coles (1657)

the old name might mean "rays of the sun" rather than "teeth of the lion"? In any case the Chinese, who have long used the dandelion, have even better names for it: two are "yellow-flowered earth-nail" and "golden hairpin weed."

### Use dandelion for...
It is high in minerals, especially potassium, and vitamins A, B, C, and D. The young leaves boiled up into a tea or eaten fresh in salads are detoxifiers, clearing blood and lymph by increasing elimination through the kidneys and bowels. This in turn benefits overall health.

If dandelion says "think spring," it also suggests "think liver." It has

a reputation as a safe liver herb, especially where there are toxins and heat in the blood. The plant's chemicals cause the gallbladder to contract, releasing bile, stimulating the liver to produce more.

Liver-related conditions aided by dandelion include jaundice and hepatitis, gallstones and urinary tract infection, painful menopause, PMT, and menstruation; improvements are achievable in the pancreas, spleen, skin, and eyesight.

One monograph on dandelion lists two pages of remedies, from abscess and acne to varicose veins and venereal warts; to the author it is a "self-contained pharmacy."

It is the bitterness in dandelion leaves that makes them so good for your digestion. The bitter taste stimulates secretion of the digestive fluids, including stomach acid, bile, and pancreatic juices. Dandelion promotes the appetite, and is recommended for those who have been ill or have lost their enthusiasm for food in advanced age.

Roasted dandelion root is a well-known and caffeine-free coffee substitute. We grind the roasted root with a few pods of cardamon just before brewing; it's also tasty with cinnamon and fennel seed. The root can also be eaten as a vegetable.

The flowers don't look very edible, but they are surprisingly good eaten straight off the plant, mild

An ancient connection with man: dandelions at Avebury henge in England in April

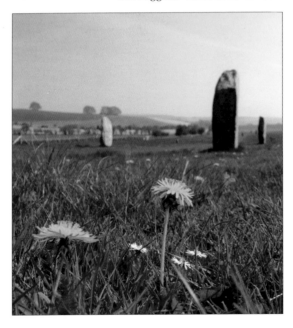

and slightly sweet. Eating a few dandelion flowers often relieves a headache too. They are delicious washed, dipped wet into flour, and fried in butter until golden brown. This needs to be a lunch dish, as the flowers only open when the sun is shining, and they are too bitter when picked in the evening.

One of Julie's first paid jobs as a girl in Jackson Hole, Wyoming, was collecting paper bags full of dandelion heads for a neighbor to make dandelion wine. This is a beautiful golden color, like distilled sunshine. The flowers also yield a refreshing dandelion "beer" and a face wash.

The sap or latex of the stems was once used in patent medicines, and was said to remove freckles and age spots, corns and warts, to help hair grow, and treat bee stings and blisters.

Dandelion is known as "piss-en-lit" in French, "pissabed" in English, and is justly renowned for its diuretic properties, that is, increasing the flow of urine. What is less familiar is how well it strengthens the urinary system. It is effective in treating bedwetting in children and incontinence in older people. All parts of the plant have this effect, but especially the leaves.

With most diuretic drugs potassium is lost from the body and has to be supplemented, but dandelion is naturally high in potassium. It can safely be used long term with-

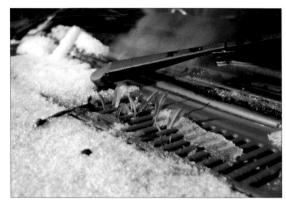

Dandelions will grow almost anywhere, from cracks in sidewalks to car hoods. They are wonderfully adaptable survivors.

out causing imbalance. The leaves boiled with vegetable peelings make a potassium-rich broth.

Dandelion's diuretic effect makes it a good herb for treating swollen ankles, for fluid retention, and high blood pressure. It can also be used to alleviate shortness of breath in the elderly.

As a medicine the whole plant is invaluable for liver and gallbladder problems, and for skin complaints including eczema and acne. Its action helps reduce high blood pressure, high cholesterol, and the pain of arteriosclerosis and joints, digestive problems, chronic illness, viral infections, and heart and lung irregularities.

Dandelion can form part of a natural cancer treatment, and taken regularly as a food and medicine may help prevent some cancers, especially breast cancer, and other chronic illnesses by keeping the body clean, toned, and healthy.

*Dandelions may well be the world's most famous weed. ... Up until the 1800s, [American] people would actually pull the grass out of their yards to make room for dandelions and other useful "weeds" such as chickweed, malva, and chamomile.*
*– Mars (1999)*

**DANDELION SAP**
- warts
- calluses
- corns
- rough skin

### Dandelion tincture

The root or the leaves can be tinctured separately for specific uses, but for general use we prefer to use the whole plant. Dig up **dandelion plants**, wash the dirt off and remove any dead leaves. The plants can be left whole or chopped up. Place in a jar large enough to hold them, and pour enough **vodka** in to cover the plants completely.

Put the jar in a cool place out of sunlight. If you chop up your plants, the tincture can be ready in as little as two weeks, otherwise leave it for a month before straining, squeezing the residue in a jelly bag or piece of muslin to get all the liquid out. Pour it into clean amber or blue glass bottles, label, and store until needed.

**Dandelion salad**
• sluggish liver
• constipation
• urinary problems
• fluid retention

**Dandelion tincture**
• skin problems
• sluggish liver
• constipation
• urinary problems
• fluid retention
• arthritis
• gout
• hangovers
• chronic illness

### Dosage
• For general health maintenance, take half a teaspoonful twice daily.
• For acute skin eruptions, take 10 drops in water frequently throughout the day until the skin clears.
• For digestive problems, recuperation from chronic illness, sluggish liver, arthritis, gout, eczema, and psoriasis, take half to 1 teaspoonful three times daily in water.
• For overindulgence in food or drink, take 10 drops in water every hour until you are feeling better.

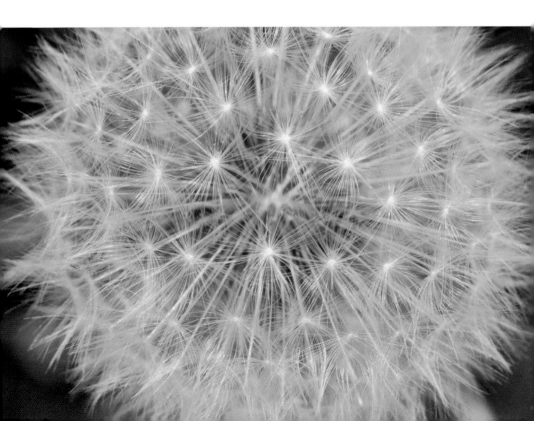

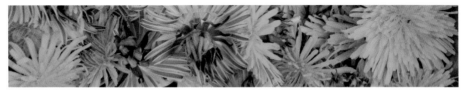

## Dandelion flower beer

Pick 100 **dandelion flowers**. Boil 4 pints of **water** with three and a half ounces of **light brown sugar** until the sugar has dissolved. Allow to cool until tepid, then pour over the dandelion flowers in a large container. Add **a lemon**, finely sliced.

Cover the container with a clean cloth and set aside in a cool place for three or four days, stirring occasionally. Strain and pour into tightly corked bottles. The beer will be ready to drink in just a few days.

## Dandelion flower infused oil

Pick enough **dandelion flowers** to fill a clean, dry jam jar. Pour in **extra virgin olive oil** slowly, allowing it to seep down around the flowers until the jar is full and there are no air pockets left.

Cover the jar with a piece of cloth held in place with a rubber band, and put the jar in a warm sunny place. It can be left outdoors during the day if the weather is clear, and brought in at night, or left on a sunny window ledge. The cloth cover lets any moisture escape. You may need to prod the flowers down to keep them immersed in the oil, as they can go moldy if left in the air.

After a week or two, or when the flowers are limp and have lost their color, strain off the oil. If you put the flowers in a cloth or jelly bag to squeeze out the oil you may get some juice as well, so you'll need to let the oil stand for a while in a jug. This will allow any water to sink to the bottom. The oil can then be carefully poured off into bottles, leaving the watery bits at the bottom of the jug.

Dandelion flower oil is an excellent rub for muscle tension and cold, stiff joints. It is good for dry skin, and can be rubbed into the delicate skin around the eyes. Don't forget this oil can be eaten too, adding a taste of sunshine to salads and other foods.

For external use, you can add essential oils to your home-made flower oil, using up to 20 drops per 3 fl oz of oil. The essential oils act as a natural preservative, and bring their own healing qualities to the mixture. Lavender, ylang ylang, and rosemary all combine well with dandelion.

**DANDELION FLOWERS**
**Flower infused oil**
- muscle tension
- muscle aches
- stiff necks
- arthritis

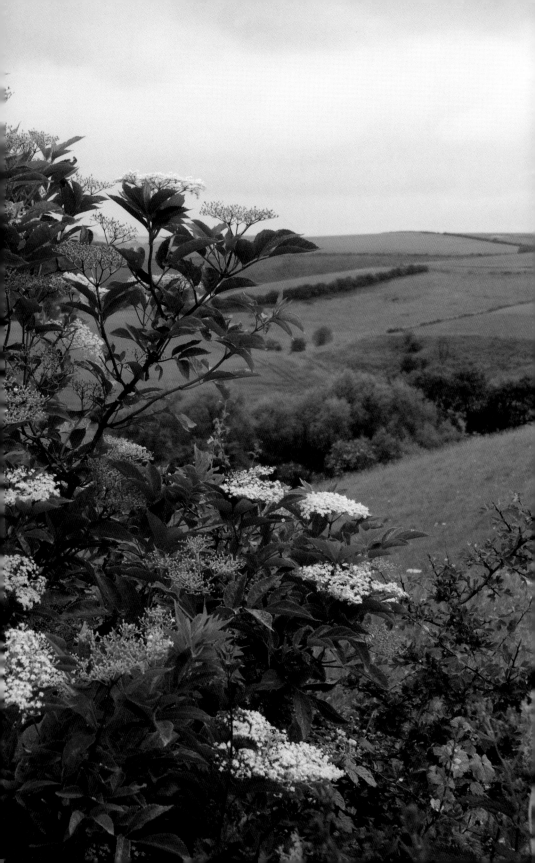

# Elder *Sambucus nigra*

**If ever the soul of a plant has been fought for, it is elder. An important herb through the ages, it has been described as a whole medicine-chest in one plant. Less used now than formerly, its flowers remain a wonderful fever remedy and delicious in drinks or desserts. The berries work against flu and colds, and help relieve coughs. The leaves, as an ointment, are good for bruises.**

Few plants are as steeped in folklore, legend and superstition as the elder. Its hollow stem was said to have been used by Prometheus to bring fire to man from the gods, and the Saxon *aeld* ("fire") may have given elder its name. The same empty stem was a ready-made flute, and the species name *sambucus* was chosen by Linnaeus for a flute made of elder.

Elder was faerie and pagan. If you were in the company of the tree on Midsummer night you would see the Faery King ride by. Another version of our name "elder" was from Hylde Moer, the elder or earth mother – when an elder planted itself in your garden it meant the mother had chosen to protect your house from lightning and your cattle from harm. You must never cut down an elder or burn it, because the mother was present, without asking her leave.

So entrenched was the cult of the elder mother that the Church vilified elder with its most powerful negative associations: Christ was said to have been crucified on an elder tree and Judas to have hanged himself on one.

And if that seemed to stretch credulity, judging by the tree's weak branches, there was something else: God had cursed elder by making its once large black berries small and its straight branches twisted. Such sanctioned hostility was borne out in a verse on elder quoted by Robert Chambers in his *Popular Rhymes of Scotland* (1847):

*Bour-tree, bour-tree, cookit rung,*
*Never straight, and never strong,*
*Ever bush and never tree*
*Since our Lord was nailed t'ye.*

Its rank smell has always been held against elder. The leaves were once sold as a fly repellent, and it was bad luck to have the flowers indoors. A rhyme went:

*Hawthorn blooms and elderflowers*
*Fill the house with evil powers.*

The plant was redolent of sex and death, the greatest taboos, yet a

**Caprifoliaceae**
**Honeysuckle family**

**Description:** A shrub or small tree, with fragrant clusters of creamy white flowers in summer, followed by black berries in fall.

**Habitat:** Hedgerows, riverbanks, woods, and waste ground.

**Distribution:** Native to Europe, introduced to North America.

**Related species:** American black elder is now considered a sub-species (*Sambucus nigra* spp.*canadensis*), as is blue elder (*S. nigra* spp. *caerulea*). They can be used interchangeably with black elder, but the raw fruit may be more likely to cause stomach upset in some people. The North American red-berried elder (*S. racemosa*) has been used medicinally but the berries are more likely to cause digestive upsets (especially the seeds of raw berries).

**Parts used:** Flowers and berries; leaves externally.

(opposite) Elder flowering in the English Lincolnshire Wolds in late June

*If the medicinal properties of its leaves, bark, berries &c. were thoroughly known, I cannot tell what our countrey-men could ail, for which he might not fetch a remedy from every hedge, either for sickness, or wound.*
– Evelyn (1664)

*What says my Aesculapius? my Galen? my heart of Elder?*
– Shakespeare, *Merry Wives of Windsor,* II.3.1126.

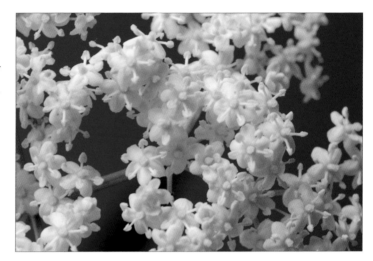

Puritan like John Evelyn could see beyond this to its medicinal virtues: "though the leaves are somewhat rank of smell and so not commendable in sallet, they are of the most sovereign virtue." An extract of the berries would "assist longaevity" and was "a kind of *catholicon* against all infirmities whatsoever … every part of the tree being useful."

The battle for control of elder has always swung like this. It was a tree of life, yet a devil's tree; it was needed, hence a good herb in the monastery garden; it was feared, so it was a witch's plant.

Yet survive it has, in town and country alike, on any patch of waste ground. Of all the wild plants in this book elderflower is the one harvested for commercial use, for cordials and other drinks.

Elderflower drinks are also widely made at home, and drug stores often run out of citric acid during the elderflower season!

Strangely, the berries are often ignored as food these days, but they make a lovely wine and are delicious cooked with apples (and were once widely used to adulterate wine and true ports).

### Use elder for...
Elder blossom is one of the best herbs for encouraging sweating to break a fever, when drunk as a hot tea, as Julie recalls:

"I was visiting my parents once in Namibia when my mother came down with a slight fever. I had seen an elder blooming in a nearby park, so dosed her with a tea of the fresh flowers before tucking her in bed. The elder worked so well that she became drenched in sweat and thought she had malaria. But a blood test was clear."

The flower tea "clears the channels" in the body, promoting elimination via the skin and the urinary tract, and supporting the circulation. Elderflowers cut congestion and inflammations of the upper respiratory tract, and break up catarrh. They reduce the symptoms of hayfever, often used with nettle tops.

Elderflower products are also used internally and externally to help clean the skin. A distilled water of the flowers made an eyewash in the 1600s, helped remove freckles and spots, and was used to cool sunburn; it will still work today.

Elderberries are well known for reducing the length and severity of colds and flu, and can be used to help prevent infection. They are an excellent winter standby.

**Cautions:** Do not eat the leaves. Some books say elderberries are toxic and shouldn't be eaten raw. This refers to the seeds of the red-berried elders, and does not appear to be true for black elder, though some people may suffer from digestive upsets. Elderberries can cause diarrhea if eaten raw in large quantity, but as a food they are more usually cooked. In a tincture or glycerite the seeds are strained out.

## Elder leaf ointment
Warm half a pint **extra virgin olive oil** in a small pan and add a couple of handfuls of chopped **elder leaves**. Simmer gently until the leaves are crisp, then strain. Return the oil to the pan. Melt 1 oz **beeswax** in the oil, then pour into ointment jars. Leave to cool and set before putting the lids on and labeling. Use for bruises, sprains, and chilblains.

## Harvesting elderflowers
Pick elderflowers on a dry sunny day, choosing those that smell lemony and fresh. In damp weather or in shady places the flowers can have an unpleasant smell. Pick the whole head of flowers. If you are drying them for tea, spread the heads on brown paper to dry, and then use a fork to strip the blossoms off the stems.

## Elderflower tea
This can be made with fresh flowers, but as their season is relatively short, the dried flowers are usually used.

Use 1 heaped teaspoonful of **dried flowers** per cupful of **boiling water.** Cover and allow to infuse for 3 to 5 minutes. Strain and drink hot and frequently for the early stages of a cold or fever, to promote sweating. For this, it combines well with equal parts of yarrow and mint. For hayfever, use in combination with nettle leaves.

Drink cold for its diuretic effect and for menopausal hot flashes, or use as a face wash.

**ELDER LEAF
Ointment**
• bruises
• sprains
• chilblains

**ELDERFLOWER
Hot tea**
• fevers
• colds and flu
• promotes sweating
• use in bath
• hay fever

**Cold tea**
• night sweats
• promotes urination
• hot flashes
• fluid retention
• use as a face wash

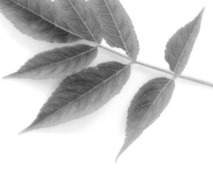

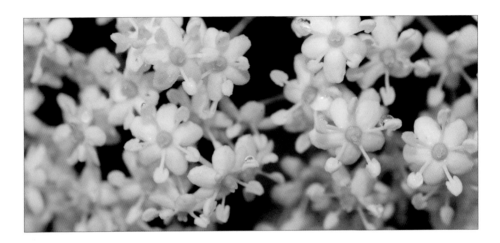

**ELDERFLOWER**
**Glycerite**
• sore throats
• stuffy noses
• hot flashes
• face lotion

**Cordial**
• hot flashes
• colds
• sore throats

**For a cold**
*Elder flowers dry boyled in milk & drink it at night. It weill sweat & do much good.*
– Book of culinary recipes 1739–79

### Elderflower glycerite

Pack heads of **elder blossom** into a large jar, then fill with **vegetable glycerine**, stirring to release any air bubbles. Put the lid on and place the jar in a warm place, on a sunny window ledge, or by a range cooker, and leave for two weeks. Strain using a jelly bag or a press. Bottle the liquid, label, and store in a cool dark place. You can use this glycerite as is, or add elderberries in the fall (see next page).

**Dose:** 1 teaspoonful as needed for sore throats. For a clear complexion and smooth skin, mix half and half with rosewater and use freely as a face lotion.

### Elderflower cordial

Pick 30 heads of **elderflower** on a dry sunny day, choosing those that smell lemony and fresh.

Boil **2 lbs sugar** in **4 pints of water** for about 5 minutes in a large sauce-pan. Pour into a large ceramic bowl and add **2 oz citric acid**, a **chopped lemon** and a **chopped orange.**

Add the **elderflower heads** and stir well. Cover with a clean cloth and leave for 4 days, stirring every day. Strain through a jelly bag and bottle. For long-term storage, the cordial can be frozen.

To drink, dilute to taste with cool sparkling water. It can also be made with hot water to encourage sweating in colds and fevers.

### Harvesting elderberries

Pick bunches of elderberries when they are ripe and black but still firm and shiny. The easiest way to strip them from their stems is to use a fork.

### Elderberry glycerite

Fill a large jar with **elderberries**, and pour in **vegetable glycerine** or elderflower glycerite to fill the gaps until the jar is full. Place in a warm spot, on a sunny window ledge, or by a range cooker, and leave for two weeks. Strain and squeeze the juice out of the berries, using a jelly bag or a press. Bottle the liquid, label, and store in a cool dark place.

This can be used on its own for coughs and sore throats or mixed with cherry bark syrup (see page 25).

### Elderberry syrup

Put **ripe elderberries** into a large saucepan with half their volume of **water**. Simmer and stir for 20 minutes. Allow to cool, then squeeze out the juice using a jelly bag or fruit press.

Measure the juice, and for every pint of juice add half pound **muscovado sugar**, a **stick of cinnamon**, a few **cloves** and a few **slices of lemon**. Simmer for 20 minutes, then strain and pour while hot into sterilized bottles.

**Dose:** Take 1 teaspoonful neat every few hours for colds and flu, or use it as a cordial and add boiling water to taste for a hot drink.

**ELDERBERRY**
**Glycerite**
• coughs
• colds
• flu

**Syrup**
• coughs
• colds
• flu

*… To press and make their eldern berry wine/ That bottled up becomes a rousing charm/ To kindle winters icy bosom warm/ That wi its merry partner nut brown beer/ Makes up the peasants christmass keeping cheer.*
– John Clare, "October," *The Shepherd's Calendar* (1827)

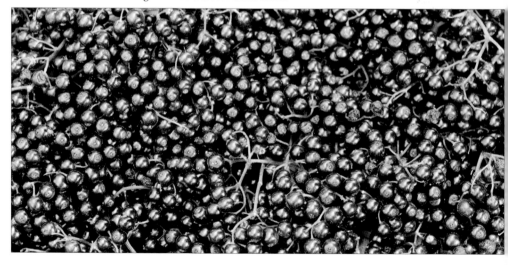

# Guelder rose, Crampbark

*Viburnum opulus*

Guelder rose is able to relieve muscle tension, both in skeletal muscles and in the smooth muscle of the intestines, lungs, and uterus. It is used on its own for cramps and muscle spasms, including uterine cramps, back pain, fibromyalgia, and irritable bowel syndrome, and in formulae for high blood pressure, arthritis and nervous tension.

**Caprifoliaceae
Honeysuckle family**

**Description:** A large shrub or small tree with palmate leaves, white blossoms and vivid red berries.

**Habitat:** Woodlands, damp places, and scrubland.

**Distribution:** Native to Eurasia and North America.

**Related species:** There are around 150 species in the genus worldwide. Black haw (*V. prunifolium*) from the eastern USA has similar herbal uses.

**Parts used:** Bark, harvested while the tree is in leaf.

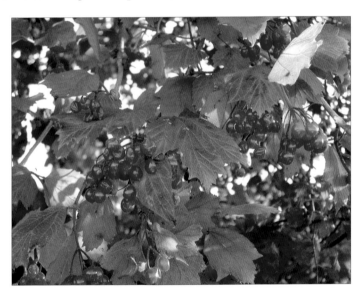

This beautiful native tree should be more widely planted in gardens for its all-year generosity. It has showy creamy-white flowerheads in early summer, while in late summer and fall the berries ripen to a stunning scarlet, their translucence lending them a gorgeous glow, and the foliage colors intensify as the weather cools. The berries are edible, and make a delicious jelly.

And if you need more reasons to grow Guelder rose, there are all the medicinal uses of the bark!

Luckily, it is also a common tree in damp woodlands and hedgerows. It has been used medicinally for centuries (Chaucer mentions it), and the name could derive from the town of Guelders, on the former German–Dutch border. Another possibility comes from its superficial similarity to elder, in the same family, reflected in the old common names water elder and white elder. Gerard calls it rose elder or Gelders rose. Crampbark is a more recent name, which well captures its principal use today.

Guelder rose really helps in rheumatic conditions where the pain is from tension rather than inflammation, easing the pain and improving blood flow to the affected area. It is a great remedy to take at the first onset of both migraines and tension headaches, and by relaxing the blood vessels it helps with high blood pressure, Raynaud's syndrome, restless legs, cramps, and menstrual pain.

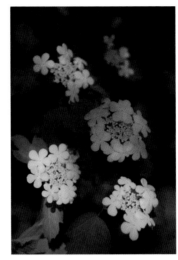

Guelder rose: The small yellowish flowers in the center are fertile while the large white flowers surrounding them are sterile.

**Decocted Guelder rose tincture**

- cramps
- menstrual pain
- headache
- muscle spasm
- backache
- spastic constipation
- IBS
- high blood pressure
- restless legs
- rheumatic pain
- Raynaud's syndrome
- poor circulation in hands and feet

*... possibly one of the best herbs known for preventing miscarriage due to stress and anxiety, and is specifically used for relaxing the uterine muscles ... among my favorite remedies for menstrual cramps.*
– Gladstar (1993)

*... will speedily quiet the uneasiness and relieve the pains of uterine and abdominal cramps and is a remedy for nervous disorders and spasms of all kinds.*
– Dr Christopher (1996)

## Harvesting Guelder rose

Guelder rose bark can be harvested any time of year, but is usually harvested in the spring or early summer. Use a small knife to remove the bark in short strips, taking care not to take too much from any branch and not to ring the limb, or it will die. The bark can be used fresh, or dried for later use.

## Decocted Guelder rose tincture

Put the pieces of **bark** you have harvested in a small saucepan, and add enough **water** to just allow them to float. Bring to a boil, then turn down the heat and simmer gently for 10 minutes. Leave to cool, then strain off the liquid. Measure it, add an equal amount of **vodka** and pour into a jar with the bark pieces you've just boiled. If you are making the tincture in the fall, you can add a few ripe berries to the jar too. Keep the jar in a cool dark place for a month, shaking it every day if you can remember.  Strain off the liquid, bottle and label.

**Dose:** Half to 1 teaspoonful in water, two to three times a day. For acute conditions, you can add 3 tsp to a glass of water and sip frequently. The tincture can also be used as a liniment rub for aching muscles.

# Hawthorn *Crataegus monogyna, C. laevigata (syn. C. oxyacantha)*

**Rosaceae
Rose family**

**Description:** Thorny shrubs or small trees with clusters of white or pink flowers in spring followed by deep red berries in the fall.

**Habitat:** Hedgerows, scrub, and woodland margins.

**Distribution:** Throughout Europe, introduced to North America and Australia. Hawthorn (*C. monogyna*) is the more common species in Britain. Midland hawthorn (*C. laevigata*) is known as smooth hawthorn in North America. They can be used interchangeably. The pink and red flowering hawthorns found in gardens and parkland are generally varieties of Midland hawthorn.

**Related species:** There are over 200 species worldwide, found in northern temperate regions. Several of these are planted as ornamentals in parks and gardens. Chinese haw (*C. pinnatifidia*) is used in Chinese medicine to calm the spirit.

**Parts used:** Flowering tops, leaves, and ripe berries.

Hawthorn is a superb heart and circulatory tonic, protecting and strengthening the heart muscle and its blood supply. It improves blood circulation around the body, and can be used to treat a wide range of circulatory problems.

Hawthorn also affects the emotional side of what we think of as "heart," by calming and reducing anxiety, helping with bad dreams and insomnia, and smoothing menopausal mood swings.

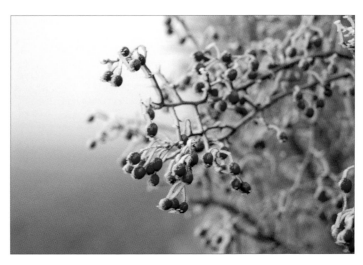

Hawthorn is *the* hedgerow plant of the British Isles. It is the most commonly found species in hedges and spinneys, both historically and in present planting; its very name means "hedge-thorn." It bounds fields and keeps stock in, it grows steadily, is readily plashed and managed, survives poor soils and high winds, and was long a sacred, protective presence.

Hawthorn is well known today as an herbal remedy for the heart and circulation, but this is a relatively new use of the plant. Old European herbals mainly talk of hawthorn for "the stone" and for drawing out thorns and splinters, and an occasional use for treating gout and insomnia. It's perhaps surprising that it wasn't thought of for the blood, because the berries are such

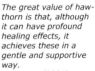

a deep blood-like color, and color was often taken as an indication of healing possibilities. Anne Pratt's mid-Victorian survey of British flowering plants (1857) expressed a conventional, and what could be called a pre-modern, view of hawthorn's value:

*The chief use of the Hawthorn is for those green impenetrable hedges which bound our meadows and lanes, which are so hardy that they are not even killed by the sea breeze, and which when whitened by their flowers are one of the greatest beauties of the rural landscape…*

The modern tale of hawthorn (there are many ancient ones too) begins with a Dr Green in County Clare, Ireland, in late Victorian times. The doctor had singular success in treating heart disease, but refused to divulge the secret of his medicine. When he died, in 1894, his daughter disclosed that he had been using a tincture of ripe hawthorn berries.

Dr JC Jennings of Chicago wrote up the story for the *New York Medical Journal* in 1896, and the use of hawthorn tincture for a variety of heart problems quickly caught on on both sides of the Atlantic.

Here is a case history recorded by another Dr Jennings, this time MC, and published in *A Treatise on Crataegus* in 1917. It is suggestive of the high esteem in which some doctors had soon come to hold hawthorn for heart treatments:

*Mr B., aged 73 years. I found him gasping for breath when I entered the room, with a pulse rate of 158 and very feeble; great oedema of lower limbs and abdomen. A more desperate case could hardly be found.*

*I gave him fifteen drops of* Cratae-gus *in half a wineglass of water. In fifteen minutes the pulse beat was 126 and stronger, and breathing was not so labored. In twenty-five minutes pulse beat 110 and the force was still increasing, breathing much easier.*

*He now got ten drops in same quantity of water, and in one hour from the time I entered the house he was, for the first time in ten days, able to lie horizontally on the bed. I made an examination of the heart and found mitral regurgitation from valvular deficiency, with great enlargement.*

This clinical success would have been a surprise to earlier generations of doctors and herbalists, as well as to contemporaries. Hawthorn had always had a mixed reputation in popular lore, and for it to be a demonstrably useful heart herb was unexpected.

There is something exciting about wild plants that have white spring flowers and dark berries in the fall. Both elder and hawthorn were fertility symbols of pre-Christian British peoples, and both plants were long ago absorbed by the incoming religion.

Hawthorn was appropriated as forming Christ's crown of thorns

*The great value of hawthorn is that, although it can have profound healing effects, it achieves these in a gentle and supportive way.*
*– Conway (2001)*

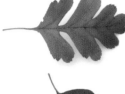

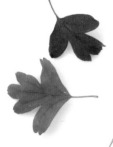

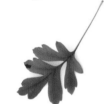

and as being the "burning bush" seen by Moses. The Glastonbury thorn was the best known of the English holy hawthorns.

In its old name of May, hawthorn was the very plant of May Day's plaited crowns and the maypole, much tamer echoes of earlier rites; yet this abundant, fertile spring plant was and still sometimes is unlucky to bring into the house.

Perhaps it was the smell of the flowers, which gives some people hayfever or was said to have lingered from the Great Plague of London; it was also reminiscent of the taboos, of death and putrefaction, but also of sex. On the other hand, an old proverb gave a softer view of hawthorn's erotic power:

*The fair maid who, the first of May,/ Goes to the fields at break of day,/ And washes in dew from the hawthorn tree,/ Will ever after handsome be.*

### Use hawthorn for...
Long the plant of the heart in folklore, we know now that hawthorn works in several ways as a restorative of the physical heart. It has the wonderful capacity to dilate the coronary arteries and strengthen the heart muscle without raising blood pressure or increasing the beat.

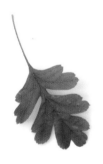

The berries, leaf, and flowers can be used to treat angina, enlargement of the heart from overwork or excessive exercise, and heart damage from over-use of alcohol.

It is important to state that heart disease is a life-threatening illness, and should be treated under the advice of a primary healthcare practitioner – your doctor or a qualified professional herbalist. If you are taking beta-blockers, only use hawthorn under supervision.

Unlike digitalis and numerous commercial preparations, hawthorn is a prophylactic with few side effects. It can – and we'd say should – be made part of personal regime to forestall future problems with the heart and circulation.

Hawthorn lowers high blood pressure and helps dissolve cholesterol and calcium deposits, making it good for arteriosclerosis, or hardening of the arteries, and plaquing.

When a fatty plaque comes loose from an artery wall it can rapidly lead to a blockage. If the artery involved is the coronary artery, which feeds the heart muscle, this blockage will mean a heart attack; if a plaque blocks an artery in the brain, it will cause a stroke. Arteries anywhere in the body can be affected, but problems often go unnoticed.

Hawthorn is also an effective treatment for intermittent claudication, where the blood vessels of the legs aren't supplying enough oxygen to the muscles, resulting in pain on walking. Similar conditions, such as Buerger's disease and Raynaud's disease, also benefit from hawthorn's gentle effects.

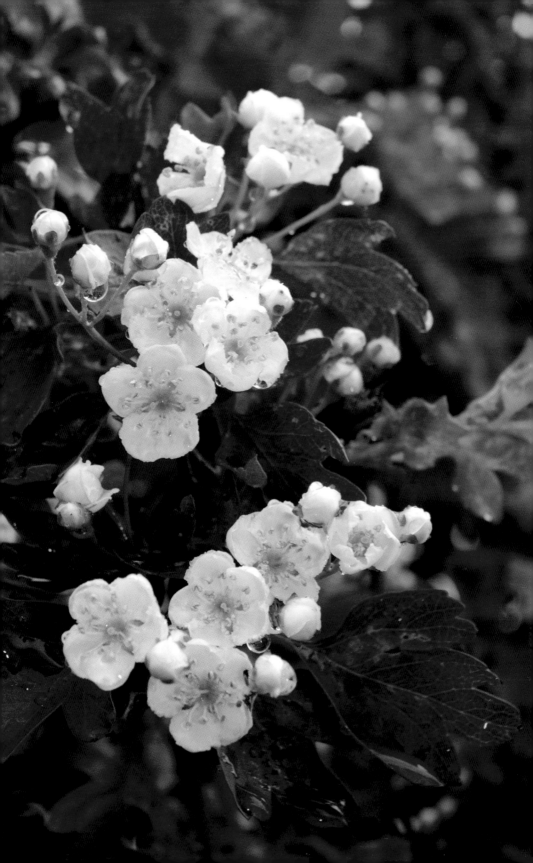

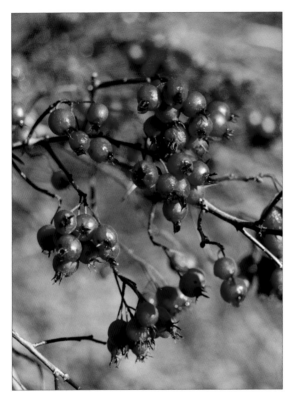

Hawthorn enhances the functioning of the heart and circulation during exercise, and taken in moderation can improve athletic performance. Also, the flavonoid compounds called procyanidins found throughout the plant help normalize blood pressure. So, if blood pressure is too high, hawthorn will lower it, and if too low it will stimulate the heart rate and raise it.

Taking hawthorn calms the spirit, and gives good results in menopausal mood swings, restlessness, and anxiety; it will quieten overactive children who have ADHD.

Hawthorn combines well with yarrow when there is constriction of the blood vessels and a risk of thrombosis or clotting. As a general heart and circulatory tonic, it is used alongside ramsons or garlic, and ginger. If the circulation needs stimulating, take it with horseradish. To improve the peripheral circulation of the limbs, use hawthorn with lime blossom.

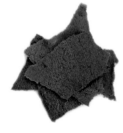

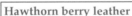

**Hawthorn berry leather**
Pick ripe **hawthorn berries** and place in a saucepan with half their volume of **water**. Simmer gently for about 15 minutes and allow to cool. Blend the mixture briefly to loosen the pulp from the seeds or mash it with a potato masher, then rub the pulp through a coarse sieve.

Pour this strained pulp into baking trays so that it is less than a quarter-inch thick, and put the trays in an oven at the lowest temperature setting to dry. If you have a food dehydrator, you can put the fruit leather trays in that, following the manufacturer's instructions. Leave until the pulp is dry and leathery and can be peeled off the trays without being sticky. Cut up and store in airtight jars. Eat about a 1 inch square every day to help keep your heart and circulation healthy.

### Hawthorn berry syrup

Put 1 lb **berries** in a large saucepan with 1 pint **water**, and slowly bring to a boil. Mash a little with a potato masher. Turn off the heat and leave to stand overnight. Bring to a boil again, then turn down the heat and simmer gently. The berries quickly lose their deep red color and turn a dingy sort of yellow. Don't worry if the decoction smells somewhat fishy at this point – the syrup will not taste like it smells.

When the mixture has sweated down to half its volume, allow to cool and then squeeze out the juice. Weigh the juice and put back into the saucepan with an equal weight of **sugar**. Bring rapidly to a boil, then pour while still warm into sterilized bottles. The finished syrup often has a strawberry-like flavor. You can use honey instead of sugar for this syrup, but the honey version does not keep as well.

**Dose:** 1 teaspoonful daily as a heart tonic or use as a flavoring.

### Hawthorn tincture

The best hawthorn tincture is made in two parts, using the flowers and leaves gathered in spring and then adding the berries in the fall when they are ripe.

**In spring:** Gather the **flowering tops** when the blossom is fresh. Remove any large twigs, and pack into a jar. Fill the jar with **vodka**, put the lid on and shake the jar to remove any air bubbles. Put the jar in a cupboard for about a month, until the blossom and leaves have lost their color, then strain off the liquid and bottle it.

**In fall:** Put the **berries** in a blender with enough **hawthorn flower tincture** to cover (if you don't have enough, you can add **vodka**), and blend to a mush. Pour the mixture into wide-mouthed jars  – this is important because hawthorn berries have so much pectin that the whole mixture will set solid, and you'll find it impossible to get it out of a narrow-necked bottle. Leave the jars in a cool dark place for a month, then poke a knife into the jar to chop the contents enough to get them out. Squeeze the liquid out using a jelly bag – this is good exercise! If you have a juice press, use that as it will be a lot less work.

Bottle and label your tincture. This will keep for several years, although it's best to make a fresh lot every year if you can.

**Dose**: 1 teaspoon once a day as a general tonic; 1 teaspoon three times a day or as advised by your herbalist for circulatory problems.

**BERRIES**
**Hawthorn fruit leather**
• heart tonic
• circulatory tonic

**Hawthorn berry syrup**
• heart tonic
• hardening of the arteries
• abnormal blood pressure
• mild angina
• anxiety, restlessness

**FLOWERS, LEAVES & BERRIES**
**Hawthorn tincture**
• heart tonic
• hardening of the arteries
• abnormal blood pressure
• palpitations
• irregular heart beat
• mild angina
• anxiety, restlessness
• intermittent claudication

**Caution:** Only take hawthorn alongside beta-blockers and other cardiovascular drugs if you are under the professional supervision of an herbal or medical practitioner.

# Honeysuckle, Woodbine *Lonicera periclymenum*

**Honeysuckle is esteemed for its superb scent and lovely flowers but should also be valued as a cooling herb. It has benefits for menopausal hot flashes, flu, fevers, heat stroke, urinary tract infections, and other hot conditions. The flowers have similar qualities to aspirin and are strongly antiseptic, being effective against a range of micro-organisms.**

**Caprifoliaceae
Honeysuckle family**

**Description:** A twining deciduous shrub with fragrant white, yellow, and red flowers followed by red berries.

**Habitat:** Hedges, woodland, and scrub.

**Distribution:** Native to Europe, where it is widespread. Introduced to North America.

**Related species:** There are around 180 honeysuckle species worldwide, several of which have medicinal qualities. Japanese honeysuckle (*L. japonica*) is a popular garden plant now naturalized in Australia and North America, with similar medicinal uses to woodbine.

**Parts used:** Flowers, harvested when in bloom during late spring, summer or fall.

Honeysuckle must be among the best-loved of wild and garden plants. It has the sweetest and most intoxicating of fragrances, and its attractive white, yellow, and red flowers keep on blooming through spring and summer. It forms lovely bowers that offer dappled shade around the front door of many a cottage; it is irresistible to the bees and hawk moths that pollinate it; and honeysuckle's scarlet berries in fall are a food source for many birds.

Its intertwining habit has made it the very symbol of love in many cultures. Honeysuckle flowers were once thought too dangerous to keep indoors because the scent would give forbidden thoughts to young ladies. Shakespeare knew well its mythic power, using it as an image of lovers sleeping enfolded in each other's arms in *A Midsummer Night's Dream.*

Honeysuckle was probably more common in Shakespeare's day, as England was so heavily wooded. The very old common names woodbine or woodbind recall this origin, and the twining habit.

Modern foresters are not quite so taken with the way honeysuckle twists around hazel stems, leaving permanent grooves that lower the commercial value. These twisted hazel stems, though, were once highly prized for making into twirly walking sticks that were said to help suitors win the woman of their dreams.

The Elizabethans would have been as interested in honeysuckle's medicinal properties as its beauty or romantic associations. They would not have known that its leaves and flowers are rich in salicylic acid, a compound similar to aspirin. But they would have been well aware that an infusion of the flowers or leaves was good for headaches, fevers, bronchial complaints, and rheumatism, as it is today.

Modern herbalists use the flowers over the leaves, but the bitter berries are seldom used, except for serious vomiting or diarrhea.

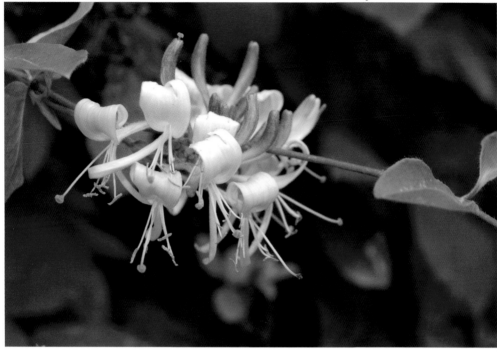

Any of the yellow-flowered varieties of honeysuckle are effective in treating heat conditions, perhaps the principal benefit of the plant today. The effect is cooling for menopausal hot flashes, fevers, sunstroke, and urinary tract infections.

Honeysuckle is also used for spasms in the respiratory system in such conditions as asthma, croup, and bronchitis. It is antiseptic and effective against many micro-organisms, reinforcing its value for sore throats and respiratory problems. A traditional Chinese formula, *shuang huang lian*, mixes honeysuckle, forsythia, and skullcap for respiratory complaints. James Duke, doyen of American herbalists, rates honeysuckle second only to eucalyptus for sore throats.

We favor the flowers steeped in honey, though a tea of the dried flowers is also good, drunk often or poured into a hot bath.

*The oyle wherein its flowers have been infused and sunned, is good against cramps, convulsions of the sinuses, and palsies and other benumming cold griefe.*
*– Parkinson (1640)*

---

**Honeysuckle flowers infused in honey or glycerine**
Pick **honeysuckle flowers** and buds and put them in a jar, then fill it up with **runny honey** or **vegetable glycerine**. Put the jar on a sunny windowsill or in another warm place and leave it for two weeks. You may need to push the flowers down into the liquid every few days to keep them covered, or they will go brown. Strain, bottle, and label.
**Dose:** 1 teaspoonful as needed for sore throats, or 3 times a day.

**Honeysuckle flowers in honey**
• sore throats
• tonsillitis
• flu
• colds
• hot flashes
• bronchitis

# Hops *Humulus lupulus*

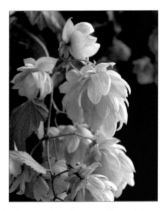

**A bitter sedative herb best known for its role in brewing and as an aid to sleep, hops also stimulate digestion and affect hormones.**

**Cannabaceae
Hemp family**

**Description:** A perennial climber, with separate male and female plants.

**Habitat:** Hedgerows, edges of woods, in gardens.

**Distribution:** Native and widespread in North America and Europe.

**Related species:** There are several subspecies of hops, and two other species are found in Asia.

**Parts used:** Female fruiting cones (strobiles).

**The medicinal use of hops preceded that in brewing, in both cases via the female flower cones, the strobiles. Used mainly in the form of a hops pillow or tincture, hops' estrogen-like compounds can reduce libido in men while increasing it in women.**

While often believed to be an introduced plant, hops are native to the British Isles. They were named *lupulus* ("small wolf") by the Romans, who wrongly thought hops strangled host plants on which they grew, like wolves strangled their prey. In Italy, hops were known as a food: the buds and tendrils still make an interesting soup, omelette, and asparagus-like boiled vegetable. Hops are rather bitter to the taste, and we think John Evelyn's opinion (1699) – "rather *Medicinal*, than fit for *Sallets*" – holds good today.

*The manifold vertues of Hops do manifest argue the wholesome-nesse of beere above ale; for the hops make it a physicall drinke to keepe the body in health, than an ordinary drinke for the quenching of our thirst.*
– Gerard (1597)

*Hops is considered by herbalists to be one of the most calming and relaxing herbs known to mankind.*
– Dewey (1996)

Hops were already cultivated for brewing in France and Germany by the eighth and ninth centuries. But ale held its place over beer in Britain until the seventeenth century; indeed, Henry VIII had banned the use of hops for a while. The Briton's ale was tradionally flavored by plants such as ground ivy (old names alehoof and tunhoof), bog myrtle, yarrow, and sage, but hops had a critical edge: all these other herbs did not preserve the brew for as long.

As beer gained ground, and hops became a commercial cash-crop in the southeast and parts of the Midlands, the plant's medicinal virtues became obscured. But then another king, George III, gave the reputation of hops a boost. His insomnia was relieved by the suggestion of his prime minister, Lord Addington, to try a hops pillow. It succeeded, and the fashion for this effective sleep aid was set. We give a recipe opposite.

Hops are now used in some 60 commercial sedative formulas in Britain, and this is the "official" use. This herb gently sedates without narcotic side effects, and soothes the smooth muscle of the stomach and bowel. It is thus a specific for nervous stomachs, IBS, and Crohn's disease. It works to relax hyperactivity in children (using half doses of hops tincture). For sleeplessness, it combines well with wood betony, vervain, skullcap, red poppy, California poppy, and passionflower. Avoid if you suffer from nervous depression.

The one fact everyone knows about hops is causing "brewer's droop" in men; less familiar is the plant's role in increasing libido in women. Both reactions relate to hops' estrogen-like compounds. Many female hop pickers used to suffer disruptions in menstruation from constant contact with the plant. But used in balance with a woman's constitution hops are a good treatment for hot flashes and in menopause. They also help control premature ejaculation in men.

As a bitter and a tonic, hops have appetite-stimulating effects that can be beneficial in cases of anorexia. They calm and relieve the spasms of irritable bowel syndrome and increase urine flow (ask any beer drinker!).

## Hops pillow
Pick **hops** strobiles (the flower cones) and dry them in a cool shady place. Make a small bag for the pillow out of **cloth**, leaving one end open – any size you like, but 8" x 10" works well. Fill the bag loosely with the dried hops (or add lavender if you wish) so that the finished pillow will be 1" thick, then stitch up the open end. Place this under your regular pillow to help with sleep.

The hops will gradually lose their volatile oils and therefore their effectiveness, so for best results replace the contents of your pillow every three months. Use hops that have been stored in the dark, in an airtight container. If your dried hops turn pinkish or reddish, their oils have been exhausted, and they should be discarded.

## Hops tincture
Pack dried **hops** cones into a jar, and fill it with **vodka**. Put the jar in a dark place for two weeks, shaking it every few days. Strain off the liquid, bottle, and label.

**Dose:** 1 teaspoonful taken in the evening to help with sleep. For menopausal hot flashes, half a teaspoonful morning and evening. For lack of appetite or sluggish digestion, a few drops pre-meals.

**Hops pillow**
• insomnia

**Hops tincture**
• hot flashes
• insomnia
• lack of appetite
• sluggish digestion

**Cautions:** Hops should not be taken if you suffer from depression. Taking hops can affect the menstrual cycle.

# Horse chestnut *Aesculus hippocastanum*

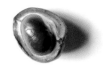

**Hippocastanaceae
Horse chestnut
family**

**Description:** A tall
tree, up to 130 ft,
with palmate leaves
in spring and huge
candelabras of white–
pink flowers in summer,
followed by conkers
in fall.

**Habitat:** Gardens,
parks, and roadsides.

**Distribution:** Native
to Asia and south-east
Europe, but widespread
as a planted and
naturalized species in
western Europe and in
eastern North America.

**Related species:** The
red horse chestnut (*A.
carnea*) is used as a
flower essence. The
North American buck-
eyes (*Aesculus* sp.) are
related, but the sweet
chestnut (*Castanea
sativa*) is not.

**Parts used:** Conkers,
collected in fall; leaves
in spring.

Familiar for its nuts, called conkers, horse chestnut is a beautiful
introduced ornamental tree. It also has significant medicinal
uses, particularly for supporting weakened veins, as in varicose
veins, hemorrhoids, and capillary fragility. It is used for
two Bach Flower Essences and in commerical quantities for
allopathic and homeopathic remedies for irregularities of the
veins. It also has some surprising other uses.

A shapely tree, with glossy brown
sticky buds in winter, lime green
hand-shaped leaves in spring, then
soft and frothy Folies-Bergère-like
pink and white flowers in summer, and hard spherical auburn
nuts, conkers, in fall – no wonder
the all-season beauty of horse
chestnut was such a hit when the
tree was introduced into England
in the early 1600s.

At first a tree of kings and owners
of great estates, it later came to
belong to everybody as Britain's
municipal tree of choice, planted
ornamentally in every avenue

and park, in every Chestnut Vil-
las of every Victorian city. Horse
chestnut trees are mainly admired
for their looks – the wood is soft
and spongy, poor for carpentry or
building.

The tree's scientific and popular
names may derive from its use in
Turkey, one of the countries of origin of the first specimens to reach
Western Europe. The Turks mixed
flour from the conkers with oats to
improve the breathing of broken-
winded horses.

Other plant historians suggest that
"horse" is meant as a derogative
comparison to the native and tasty
sweet chestnut (which is unrelated botanically). Horse chestnut
conkers do contain a complex
bitter chemical, escin (aescin in UK
spelling), as the plant's active prin-
ciple, and this is said to be toxic to
humans in very large quantities.

The tree has surprisingly varied
uses. The bark was an emergency
quinine substitute for malaria

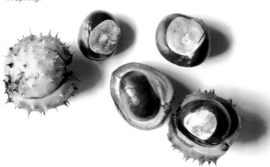

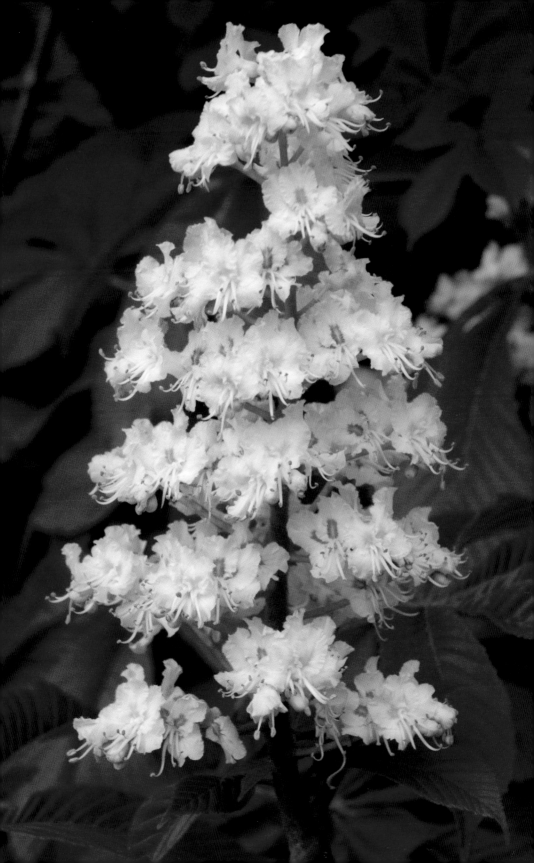

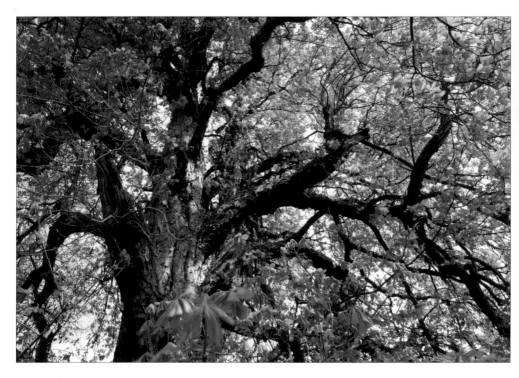

[Aescin, found in conkers] ... *reduces leakage and is used in the treatment of oedema (lower leg swelling) and has proved to be as effective as compression stockings. It strengthens and tones the blood vessels and is becoming very important in the treatment of varicose veins and chronic venous insufficiency (CVI) ... Haemorrhoids respond well too...*
– Howkins (2005)

and other fevers. The flower buds once made an ersatz flavoring for beer. Conkers produce a good soapy lather for shampoo and to clean clothes, stop mold, and repel clothes moths.

And, little known today, conkers were used for explosives during the First World War. With other sources of acetone unavailable, British children collected 3,000 tons of conkers secretly in summer 1917 (their schools received a certificate). The research chemist seconded to the government's chestnuts plan, Chaim Weizman, then in Manchester, would become first president of Israel in 1948.

Other new "explosive" chestnut issues include worries about a leaf miner moth damaging (but not killing) mature trees, and the charge that children are at risk while playing with conkers if they chew or eat them. Sadly, the game is now banned in some English schools, but it would need concerted force-feeding to reach toxic levels of escin, and the bitter taste is already off-putting to children.

### Use horse chestnut for...
Horse chestnut is a leading herbal treatment for weakened veins, including varicose veins, hemorrhoids, acne rosacea, and chronic venous insufficiency (CVI). It has

an unusual capacity to strengthen small blood vessel walls by reducing the size and number of the pores; it also works well on wrinkles by tightening the skin (an alternative to Botox, perhaps?), and for fluid retention or edema.

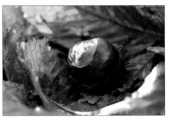

*Aesculus has unique action on the vessels of the circulatory system. The herb appears to increase the elasticity and tone of the veins while decreasing vein permeability.*
*– Hoffmann (2003)*

Horse chestnut is taken both internally as a tincture and externally as a cream, oil, or lotion. Internal use should be in small doses and under the supervision of an herbalist, in case of stomach irritation.

Commercially, it is grown for horse chestnut seed extract (HCSE) and a homeopathic remedy. It also makes two Bach Flower Essences, namely chestnut bud and white chestnut.

### Conker tincture
Collect the **conkers** as soon as they drop to the ground in early fall. They will usually come out of their green spiky husks by themselves. While fresh, they are quite soft, but they soon harden and are much more troublesome to cut. Use a serrated knife and be careful in chopping them up, as they can skid out from under the knife blade.

Put the chopped conkers in a jar and pour in enough **vodka** to cover them. Leave in a dark cupboard for a month, shaking every few days. It is normal for the alcohol to extract a milky sediment from the seeds. Strain and bottle, or use to make the lotion below.

**Internal use:** 5 drops in water twice a day, or as recommended by your herbalist.

### Horse chestnut leaf oil
Pick **leaves** in spring before the flowers open. Chop them up and put them in a jar large enough to hold them. Fill the jar with **extra virgin olive oil**. Stir to remove any air bubbles, and top up with more oil if necessary. Put on a sunny windowsill to infuse for a month, then strain off the oil into a jug. Allow this to settle for half an hour. Carefully pour the oil into jars, leaving any watery sediment behind at the bottom of the jug. Apply directly to the skin or use to make the lotion below.

### Horse chestnut lotion
Chill equal amounts of **conker tincture**, **horse chestnut leaf oil**, and **castor oil** in the fridge overnight, then blend until creamy. Bottle. Shake well before use, as it may separate on standing. Apply twice a day.

**Conker tincture**
- varicose veins
- thread veins
- fragile capillaries

**Horse chestnut leaf oil**
- varicose veins
- thread veins
- fragile capillaries

**Horse chestnut lotion**
- varicose veins
- thread veins
- fragile capillaries

**Cautions:** May cause digestive irritation when taken internally. If you are pregnant or breastfeeding, or using blood-thinning medication, only take horse chestnut under professional supervision.

# Horseradish *Armoracia rusticana*

**Brassicaceae
(Cruciferae)
Cabbage family**

**Description:** A perennial, which forms large patches. The leaves are dock-like, but bright green with parallel veins and wavy edges, and often full of holes from snails. In summer there may be trusses of white flowers.

**Habitat:** Along roadsides, on waste ground, and in kitchen gardens.

**Distribution:** Widely cultivated. Often a garden escape, it spreads by strong lateral roots, and is hard to remove once you have it.

**Parts used:** Roots.

**Horseradish root is hot and pungent, and the same qualities that make it the chosen accompaniment to roast beef also power its medicinal uses. It stimulates digestion, is an active eliminator of the waste products of fevers and colds, clears the sinuses, and is warming for rheumatism and muscle aches.**

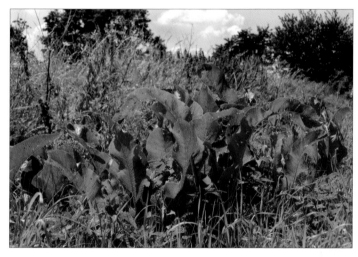

*… it is also a good remedy in strong bodies, both for the Cough, the Tissicke and other diseases of the lunges … the roote bruised and laid to the place grieved with the Sciatica-gout, jointach, or the hard swellings of the spleene and liver, doth wonderfully helpe them all.*
– Parkinson (1640)

Horseradish is this book's example of a hot, pungent, and stimulating herb. Lacking native ginger or galangal, horseradish is a good temperate heating herb, although the mustards have similar virtues.

Horseradish is a bit of a show-off, a hot cabbage originating in southern Russia, with large, coarse, wavy-edged leaves that glisten in the rain. It has small and pretty white flowers, but its main claim to fame is its long and sturdy white tap root. And this hides its healing secrets.

The root is the part that is used medicinally, as it is to make Britain's customary sauce for roast beef. We are breaking our own rules about using roots for three reasons: horseradish is abundant, if not invasive; a few roots are all you need for a year's supply as a standby medicine; and it regenerates quickly from the least fragment of root left behind.

It was a medicine long before it became a condiment, but works in a parallel way in both uses. The outer layer of root is beige and inoffensive but as soon as you cut into the tissues beneath you are assailed by a hot and biting smell that makes your eyes water.

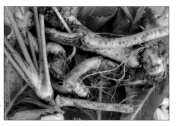

In small amounts the grated root, usually preserved in vinegar or a cream sauce, lifts the gastric enzymes into overdrive to break down the cell structure of cooked beef and prevent indigestion. Note that larger amounts can inflame the stomach lining in some people.

A mustard-like oil is being created here and released, stimulating digestive and other reactions. The mucous membranes in the mouth and throat also react immediately, and the effect is wonderful for clearing blocked sinuses.

This vigorous response accounts for the use of horseradish in promoting elimination in flus, fevers, coughs and catarrh. Be aware that it is an active process, with hot sweats and many tissues needed.

The cut root can be rubbed on stiff or aching joints and muscles to bring warmth to the skin. Rheumatic conditions can be eased using a poultice, but people with sensitive skin may react by blistering. Its antiseptic and anti-microbial qualities offer relief for boils.

Do remember the root's strength and volatility. It is not called "horse," meaning "coarse" or "rough," for nothing. An earlier English name, red cole, is said to be because the fiery taste was like red-hot coals. John Pechey noted (1707): "horseradish provokes the appetite, but it hurts the head."

**Horseradish syrup**
- coughs
- colds
- fevers
- sinus congestion

**Horseradish sauce**
- sinus congestion
- sluggish digestion

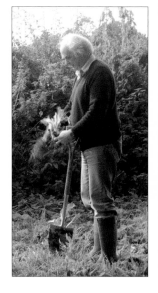

### Horseradish cough syrup

Grate a **horseradish root** into a bowl (outdoors if the fumes are strong). Whatever amount you make, cover this with **sugar.** Stir well, and leave for a few hours until a syrup develops. Strain off the liquid. If it is too fluid, heat until it reduces to the consistency you like. Pour into a bottle. It is strong, so dosage is no more than 3 tablespoons a day.

### Horseradish sauce

Chop **fresh horseradish root** and put in a blender with enough **cider vinegar** to blend. Store in the fridge. Use as a condiment, or chew a teaspoonful to clear blocked sinuses. The vinegar can be strained off after a week or two to use in the formula given on page 191.

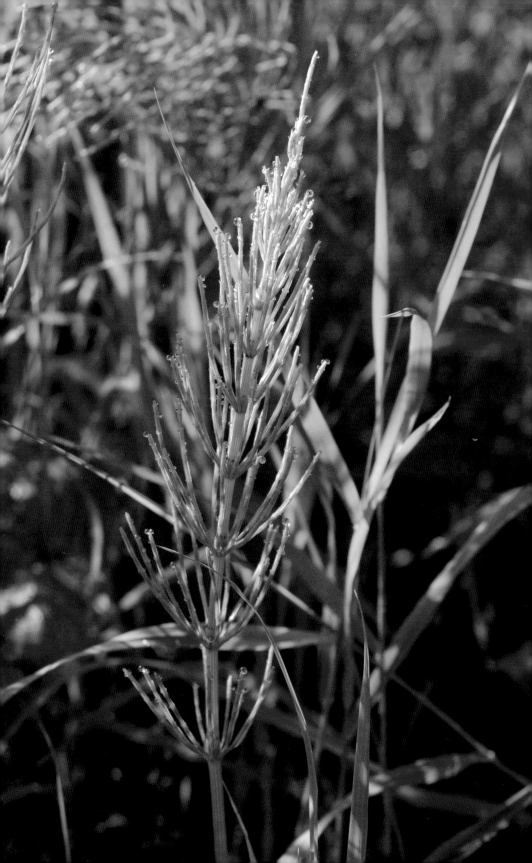

# Horsetail *Equisetum arvense*

**Horsetail is one of the oldest of plants and a long-used folk remedy for the urinary system, cystitis, incontinence, bedwetting, and prostate problems. It is the leading source of plant silica, and so helps where this mineral is deficient, as shown by symptoms like brittle nails, thin hair, and allergies. Externally, it is good for rheumatism, chilblains, and skin problems, and helps wounds, joints, and sprains to heal.**

When we say horsetail is old we do really mean old: relatives of our one foot-tall common plant grew a hundred feet tall and were the forest trees of the Carboniferous age, roughly 270–370 million years ago. You can see fossilized traces of proto-horsetail in lumps of domestic coal today, and apart from size the prehistoric and modern look uncannily alike.

The name *equisetum* refers to "horse" and "bristle," giving rise to the common English name. To the Romans it was "hair of the earth."

Horsetail is now esteemed as the main source of silica in the plant world. In effect little more than a skeleton of silica, it contains 30% or more of this element, depending on the soil; the burnt ash has over 80% silica.

Such a rich natural source of silica was recognized long ago. Old names of horsetail include pewterwort, shave-grass and bottlebrush, which hint at its ability to scour but not damage pewter, and

safely polish wood and glass. The plant was sold in London streets up to the eighteenth century for such purposes. It is said that powdered horsetail ash mixed with water is still the best silver cleaner.

Another unique quality of the plant is that it doesn't have leaves or flowers as such, and spreads by means of spores, like a fern. In spring, fertile stems grow up from deep underground rhizomes. These stems are bare with cone-like heads full of spores – "drumsticks poking out of the ground," says one author. Another writer thinks it "resembles moth-eaten asparagus." These softish stems die back and are replaced in summer by segmented, stiff and infertile stems with narrow leaves sprouting from nodes, something like pine needles on a bamboo.

While the spore stems can be eaten, and were favored by the Romans as a tonic salad, the silica-rich summer stems are better used for cleaning your pots and for their herbal qualities.

**Equisetaceae
Horsetail family**

**Description:** A leafless non-flowering perennial with hollow, jointed stems, growing up to a foot tall. It looks like a miniature Christmas tree, and has spreading green teeth on the stem sheath.

**Habitat:** Roadsides, gardens, and waste ground.

**Distribution:** Widespread in Europe, Asia, and North America. Introduced to the southern hemisphere.

**Related species:** Two other species have a traditional medicinal use: wood horsetail (*E. sylvaticum*), similar to field horsetail but more delicate and drooping at the tip; and rough horsetail (*E. hyemale*), which has no branches. The other horsetail species are not used for medicine.

**Parts used:** Aboveground parts harvested in summer.

## Is horsetail toxic?

You may have read that horsetail is toxic or that it can irritate the digestive tract.

Horsetail is toxic to livestock if they eat large quantities of it. With horses, a thiamine (vitamin B1) deficiency is caused when they eat hay contaminated with horsetail. Thiaminase, which causes this, is destroyed by heat, so is not present in a horsetail tea or syrup.

Horsetails do contain alkaloids, including palustrine, but there don't seem to be any records of toxicity in humans. We've had no experience of horsetail causing irritation when using it long-term as a tea in combination with other herbs.

It seems that horsetail would be more likely to irritate if it is taken in capsules as a powdered herb where the non-soluble silica is ingested, and yet many herbalists use horsetail in capsule form with good results. Water extracts of horsetail are unlikely to cause irritation.

To be safe: Do not eat large quantities of horsetail and avoid the species of horsetail not normally used medicinally.

## Use horsetail for...

A key virtue of horsetail is that its silica is water-soluble, meaning that it can be readily transported around the body in solution form. Taken as a tea or syrup, it reaches your nails and joints, hair, and skin; externally it makes a good poultice and hair rinse, or can be added to the bath or body lotion.

Horsetail may help if you have weak or brittle nails, thin hair with split ends, chronic cystitis or bladder irritation, multiple allergies, or weak joints and connective tissue.

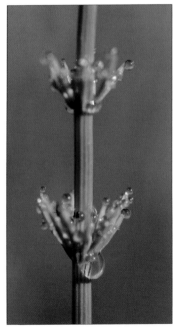

A young field horsetail (*E. arvense*) collects the early morning dew. Note the green joints, an identifying characteristic.

Horsetail can, in certain cases, work wonders in rebuilding joints and other connective tissues.

One case of horsetail's value was told by a massage therapist who thought she might have to give up her work on account of pain and weakness of the wrist joint. Taking horsetail corrected this, and indeed also led to her fingernails growing much faster. She had to cut them more often to remain a smooth operator!

There is a tradition of horsetail being used to strengthen bones and teeth, and it is often found in formulae for osteoporosis and bone fractures. It helps in the healing process after surgery.

Horsetail seems to work by strengthening the channels in the body, including the arteries and veins, and assists the free passage of fluids. One of its common names, bottle brush, probably refers to its shape but could as easily relate to this clearing of channels.

Horsetail is mildly diuretic, meaning it can clear the kidneys without exhausting them. It is useful in teas for cystitis, incontinence, and other bladder issues, and can help with the problems associated with prostate enlargement.

It is also known as a wound herb, releasing pus and damaged cells from infected wounds. Another way it works on wounds is to slow the bleeding.

## Harvesting horsetail

Pick horsetail in early summer, cutting the plant several inches above the ground so that it can grow back. For teas, dry it quickly, so that the plants don't turn brown. Crushing the plants lightly with a rolling pin helps the moisture escape. When dry, cut up into short pieces.

## Cystitis tea blend

Combine roughly equal parts by volume of dried **horsetail** and **couch-grass**, and whichever you have on hand of the following: **bilberry leaves, yarrow,** or **pellitory of the wall**.

Use a rounded teaspoonful of the mixture per mug of boiling water in a teapot, and leave to brew for 10 minutes.

**Dose:** Drink a cupful every two hours for acute cystitis, and continue with three cups a day for a while until you are completely over the cystitis.

## Horsetail tea

Add **a rounded teaspoonful of dried horsetail** and **half a teaspoonful of sugar** to **2 cups of water** in a small saucepan. Bring to a boil, turn down the heat and simmer gently, uncovered, until the liquid has reduced by about half.

**Dose:** Drink a cup occasionally to keep your skin, nails, and hair strong and healthy.

Make triple strength and add a cupful to hot baths and foot baths to help heal sprains and other injuries. It is remarkably effective.

## Horsetail syrup

This recipe keeps well, is convenient to take, and tastes good.

**A couple of handfuls of fresh horsetail (about 2 ounces)**
**1 pint water**
**three and a half ounces of sugar**

Place the ingredients together in a pan, boil, then reduce heat and simmer for half an hour until the horsetail turns dark green and becomes soft. Strain off the liquid and return it to the pan with an additional 5 oz sugar. Boil for 5 minutes, allow to cool, then bottle. Makes about 13 fl oz syrup.

**Dose:** Take one teaspoonful a day for two or three weeks, then take a break for a week before resuming if needed.

**Horsetail tea**
• cystitis
• incontinence
• bedwetting
• weak nails
• skin problems
• brittle hair
• benign prostate enlargement

**Horsetail bath**
• rheumatic pains
• skin problems
• chilblains
• sprains

**Horsetail syrup**
• incontinence
• bedwetting
• weak nails
• thin or brittle hair
• chronic cystitis
• benign prostate enlargement

*... it doth perfectly cure wounds, yea, although the sinues be cut asunder.*
– Galen (1st century AD)

*An excellent remedy, internally and external-ly, for the whole kidney and bladder system.*
– Treben (1980)

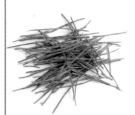

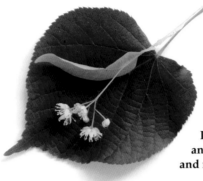

# Lime, Linden *Tilia* spp.

**The perfect remedy for stress, tension, and over-work, lime blossom helps us relax and sleep well. It soothes irritation, boosts the immune system, and protects the heart by reducing cholesterol levels and relaxing the arteries.**

**Tiliaceae**
**Lime family**

**Description:** Tall, elegant trees with deciduous, heart-shaped leaves, and fragrant flowers in summer.

**Habitat:** Woods, hedgerows, parks, and gardens.

**Distribution:** Small-leaved lime, European lime, and large-leaved lime are native to Europe, but grown in parks and gardens elsewhere. American basswood is native to North America.

**Species:** Common lime (*Tilia* x *europaea*) is the hybrid of small-leaved lime (*T. cordata*) and large-leaved lime (*T. platyphyllos*). These are the species traditionally used in Europe. American basswood (*T. americana*) can be used the same ways.

**Parts used:** Flowers, picked when the first flowers in each bunch have opened in summer.

**Linden tea is widely enjoyed in France where it is drunk as a daily beverage for its pleasant honey-like taste and its health benefits. It is also wonderful for children.**

There is nothing quite like walking under lime trees when they are in full flower in early summer, drowsily fragrant and loudly humming with the buzz of hundreds of honeybees. Bees adore lime blossom, and make a flavorsome honey from it that retains the calming effects of the flowers.

Linden's heady scent does have an uplifting effect on consciousness, and in folklore it was said that if you fell asleep under a lime tree you could wake up in fairyland. More practically, if you park your car under one in high summer, it will be covered with sticky droppings of honeydew from greenfly that live on the leaves.

The name lime can be confusing, as many of us think of lime fruit, a relative of the lemon. All that links the two is the color, which is similar in the leaves of linden trees and the citrus fruit. There is also no connection with limestone.

The blossom season is short and can easily be missed, especially if the weather is bad.

## Use lime or linden for…

Medicinally, lime blossom is best known as a calming, relaxing remedy. It can be used to treat high blood pressure, and arteriosclerosis, particularly where stress and anxiety are major factors. It is a circulatory relaxant, working to destress the arterial walls.

Relieving tension as it does, linden encourages a restful relaxing sleep, helping you wake refreshed and clear-headed. It was recommended as a sedative in Britain during the Second World War.

The tea, drunk hot, promotes sweating. This can be used to "break a fever," with sweating being the body's natural way of preventing a fever from burning too hot, while also helping eliminate toxins through the skin and clear-

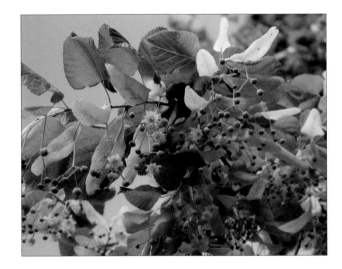

ing them through the urine. If the linden infusion is drunk cool, it is cooling to the body and useful for treating the hot flashes associated with menopause. Cold linden tea makes a delightful light summer drink on a hot day.

Linden is also warming and relaxing to the digestive sytem. It can help whenever tension goes to the digestive tract, either through eating on the run or through general anxiety. Related tension conditions, like cramps, colic, and period pains, can also be alleviated.

Being a gentle remedy with a pleasant taste, linden is particularly good for treating children. It quietly calms an overactive or fractious child, soothing and relaxing them. It is effective when they have nervous digestion or trouble sleeping, and can also be used for coughs and colds and flu, alone or with elderflower.

Externally, the tea can be rubbed into the skin to give relief in inflamed conditions such as boils, rashes, bites, scalds, and burns, or used for sore eyes. It is also soothing in a bath and or for massage.

Homeopathically, linden has much the same uses as the herb, being specific for children's toothache and women's pelvic inflammation. The inner bark of linden is known as bast (bass in the United States, giving basswood, another name for the tree). Bast can be made into a tea that is soothing for diarrhea.

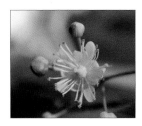

**Hot linden tea**
- nervous tension
- anxiety
- stress
- high blood pressure
- colds
- fevers and flu
- insomnia
- tension headache
- migraine

**Cold linden tea**
- hot flashes

**Linden tincture**
- nervous tension
- anxiety
- stress
- high blood pressure
- insomnia

### Linden tea

Use the new flowers and unopened buds, with their stalk and leaf sheath. Pick on a dry sunny day, and avoid any blossoms with a blackish mildew growing on them. The lime blossom season is very short, with the blossoms only at their best for about a week, so if the weather is wet during this time you are better off tincturing the blossom than drying it.

Dry the flowers out of the sun until they are crispy. Once dry, you can remove the larger stalks and store the blossom in paper bags or jars in a cool dark place. If exposed to light, lime blossom will soon deteriorate. If it turns a pinkish color, it should be discarded.

Use a heaped teaspoonful of **dried blossom** per cup of **boiling water** in a teapot, and infuse for about 5 minutes. This is a good evening drink as it will relax without being too sedative. Drink a cupful one to three times a day for anxiety or restlessness. For colds or fevers, drink small amounts of the hot tea throughout the day to soothe, clear catarrh and promote perspiration. Drink cold for hot flashes.

### Linden tincture

Fill a jar with the **freshly picked blossom**, and top it up with **vodka**. Leave it in a cupboard for two weeks, shaking every few days. Strain, bottle, and label.

**Dose:** Half a teaspoonful 2 or 3 times a day.

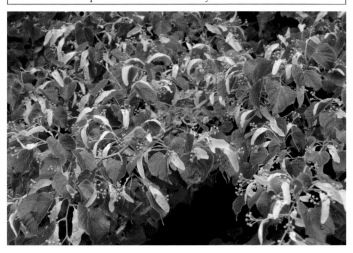

Small-leaved lime,
Bardney Woods,
Lincolnshire, June

# Lycium *Lycium barbarum, L. chinense*

**Marketed as goji berry, lycium is gaining a reputation as an exotic health food or "superfruit." It is actually naturalized in North America and Britain, known as the Duke of Argyll's tea plant, Chinese wolfberry, box thorn, or matrimony vine.**

**The berries make a rejuvenating tonic with a wide range of claimed benefits including improving eyesight and helping reduce the side effects of chemotherapy in cancer patients.**

Lycium originates in China and has been part of Chinese medicine for millennia. Its undoubted health benefits have become something of a fad in the West in the last decade or so.

In Chinese cuisine worldwide young leaves and seedlings of lycium are used for soup, and the bark of the root medicinally for malaria and high blood pressure. However, it is the tasty orange–red berries, known as *gou qi zi* (or goji), that are prized.

In Chinese terms, the berries nourish and tonify the liver and kidney meridians, and address blood and *yin* deficiency. In practice this means the berries are useful for conditions as varied as dryness, sore back and legs, weak muscles and ligaments, impotence, dizziness, and vision problems.

What may be surprising is that this plant has actually been a naturalized plant in Britain since the 1730s. The story goes that the third

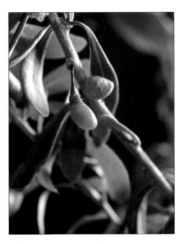

Duke of Argyll, Archibald Campbell (1682–1761), an avid plant collector, was sent a true tea plant, *Camellia sinensis*, and a lycium, but the labels were switched in the ship's hold. The name Duke of Argyll's tea plant (or tea tree) for lycium stuck and was kept even once the mistake was recognized. Other names lycium has attracted include Chinese wolfberry, box thorn, and matrimony vine.

**Solanaceae
Nightshade family**

**Description:** An arching, floppy shrub with small leaves, and purple flowers, followed by scarlet berries in the fall.

**Habitat:** Hedgerows, gardens, and near the sea, growing on a variety of soils.

**Distribution:** Native to Asia and possibly to eastern Europe. Found in most European countries and widely distributed in North America.

**Related species:** *Lycium chinense* (Chinese tea plant, Chinese desert thorn) and *L. barbarum* (Duke of Argyll's tea plant, matrimony vine) are very similar and may be used interchangeably. There are around 80 other species in the genus, found in the Americas, Eurasia and Africa.

**Parts used:** Berries gathered in fall.

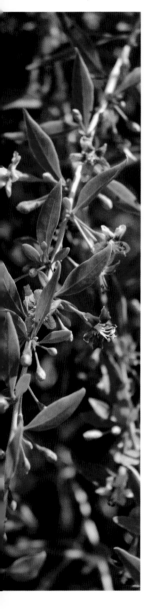

### Use lycium for…

Lycium is both a food and a medicine, and the berries can be eaten daily, dried if fresh isn't available, with claimed improvement in strength, eyesight, and male sexual performance. They are safe even in quantity, with no reported safety issues, except when somebody has problems with nightshade family plants, such as potato or tomato.

The fresh berry is tasty and somewhat astringent, resembling a small persimmon, and when dried is like a sweet red raisin. We eat dried berries on cereal or hot with rice; in China itself lycium tea, coffee, wine, and beer are all made.

There has been considerable recent hype about the "superfood" benefits of lycium taken as a juice, but we make no comment here on the claims for commercial goji products. Full-scale research is lacking, and we base our comments on our own experience and that of herbalists whose opinion we respect.

One benefit of lycium that is generally accepted is to promote a healthy gut flora, while lowering "bad" LDL and VLDL cholesterol levels in the bloodstream. The berries serve to stabilize the capillaries, veins, and arteries throughout the body. They work on thread and varicose veins, and fragile capillaries that bleed under the skin. They also help to reduce narrowing of the arteries (atherosclerosis), thereby benefiting cold hands and feet.

This effect of lycium berries on capillaries is one reason they are good for the eyes; they also contain high levels of lutein and other carotenoids needed by the retina and for healthy eye functioning.

Regular use of lycium berries can help improve night vision, reduces excessive watering of the eyes, and delays the onset of cataracts and glaucoma. The berries also stimulate lubrication of dry, red, or painful eyes, and prevent macular degeneration.

There are, further, indications that the berries enhance the beneficial effects of chemotherapy and radiation while also protecting cancer patients against the reduced white blood cell count that will often accompany these treatments. The berries support the liver against the side effects of medication and help relieve cachexia (malnutrition and other metabolic disturbances linked with cancer and AIDS). This liver protection also extends to exposure to toxic chemicals.

In addition, the berries, with plentiful antioxidants and high levels of vitamin C, reduce inflammation, enhance the immune function, and slow down tumor growth.

These are substantial and substantiated benefits for any herb, especially one that is widely naturalized. Lycium has also attracted official attention. It was specifically named in 2003 by a British government department looking

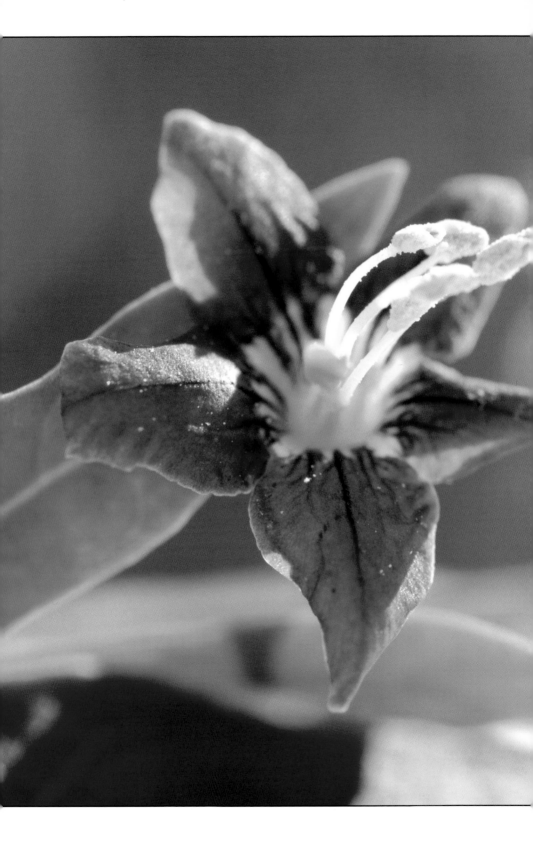

[Lycium fruit and leaf] *makes one feel happy and vigorous.*
– Lu Ji, *Shi Shu*, an ancient Chinese text

[do not eat lycium] *when traveling thousands of miles from home*
– Chinese saying, referring to sexual potency of lycium

at protecting traditional hedgerows (the locations named were in maritime Suffolk and Norfolk). More recently, in mid-2007, goji products were officially approved for sale as a food in the UK after demonstrating a proven history of use, mainly in the UK Chinese population, for many years.

In China it has long been claimed that lycium improves sexual performance, mainly in older men. Research has found that regular doses of the berries can raise testosterone levels when these are deficient. Many older men have this problem, so to this extent lycium may reduce impotence and can be seen as aphrodisiac.

Allied to the last use, lycium is renowned as anti-aging, one Chinese name being "drive-away-old-age-berries." This is good news,

but marketing claims that one man, Li Qing Yen, lived for 252 years (1678–1930) because he took daily lycium are surely excessive.

Our descriptions of lycium's many and varied "virtues," in the old herbal phrase, should not cloud the fact that it is an effective general energy-restoring tonic treatment, which can be safely taken on a long-term basis.

For example, a serving of 3.5 oz of dried berries has been estimated to supply 100% of daily needs of iron and riboflavin (vitamin B2), and nearly all the selenium and calcium. It is reasonably strong in vitamin C but exceptionally rich in polysaccharides and zeaxanthin.

Goji is not a cheap commercial product, but it need not be expensive to use if you harvest from a

Lycium in Lincolnshire: a sprawling hedge in the English village of Nettleton, in June

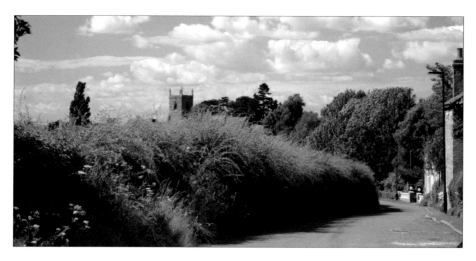

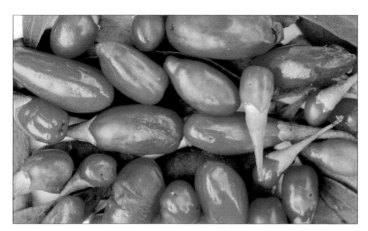

Both the berries and leaves of lycium can be eaten

local field side or plant your own lycium hedge. It is easy to grow from seed, but note that snails adore it and will devour seedlings. Once established, it is vigorous (it is used as a dune-fixer), and needs strong springtime pruning. This effort could repay you with a mass of beautiful purple flowers and brilliant scarlet berries later.

Lycium is interesting, with both ancient and very modern health applications. Goji berries and juice are a fashion of the day, with China exporting $120,000,000 of these products in 2004. But even if this commercial fad declines, lycium is worthy of a place in your garden, with much to commend it as food and medicine.

### Harvesting lycium berries
The berries are picked in the fall when they are ripe. These scarlet, glossy fruits are enjoyed by a variety of wildlife, so you will have some competition. The best ones are often found where bramble and nettle help protect them, but they have no thorns themselves. They can be eaten fresh and have an unusual flavor, similar to persimmon with perhaps a hint of red bell pepper.

### Lycium berry tincture
Put your fresh **lycium berries** in a blender with enough **vodka** to cover them, and blend briefly. Pour into a jar and leave in a cool dark place for a couple of days, then strain off the liquid. Bottle and label.

**Dose:** 1 teaspoonful 2 to 3 times a day.

**Lycium berry tincture**
- eyesight
- fragile capillaries
- varicose veins
- thread veins
- high cholesterol
- aphrodisiac
- fertility

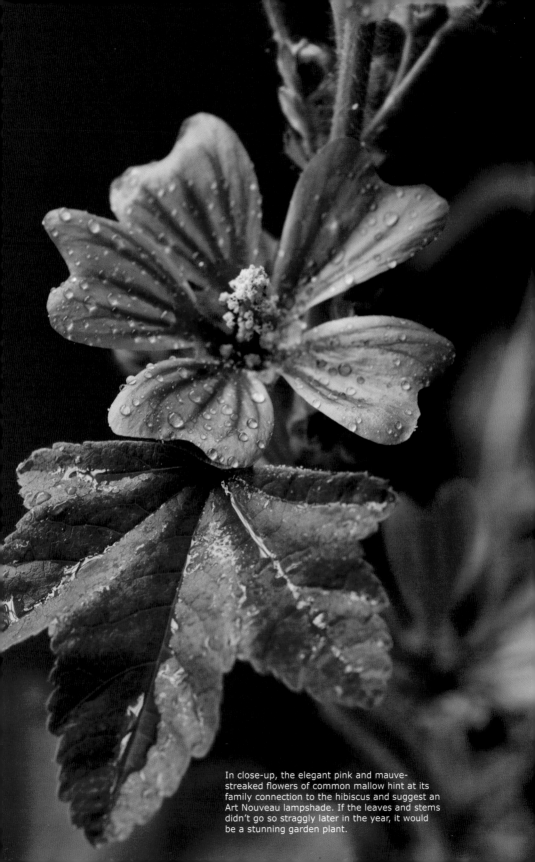

In close-up, the elegant pink and mauve-streaked flowers of common mallow hint at its family connection to the hibiscus and suggest an Art Nouveau lampshade. If the leaves and stems didn't go so straggly later in the year, it would be a stunning garden plant.

# Mallow *Malva sylvestris*

**The common or tall mallow has suffered by comparison with its more famous cousin, the marsh mallow, the only member of the family to be an "official" herb. But marsh mallow is rare as a wild plant and moreover is dug up for its root, so for the many soothing qualities of mallow, internal and external, the common form offers a highly effective alternative.**

**Malvaceae
Mallow family**

**Description:** A tall or sprawling perennial growing to 3 feet tall with pinkish-purple flowers and ivy-shaped leaves.

**Habitat:** Roadsides and bare ground.

**Distribution:** Native to Europe and northern Africa, but widespread as an introduced species in North America where it is known as tall mallow.

**Related species:** Marsh mallow (*Althaea officinalis*) is now quite rare in its native habitats but is easily grown as a garden plant.

**Parts used:** Leaves and flowers collected in summer.

The latest official list of British herbs, the *British Herbal Pharmacopoeia* 1996, describes only one mallow, the marsh mallow (*Althaea officinalis*), which has become rare in the wild in the British Isles. For commercial use it is now imported from eastern Europe. The confection "marshmallow" was once cooked from the roots of this plant but has long since ceased to be made of anything herbal.

Its abundantly found cousin, the common, high or blue mallow (*Malva sylvestris*), has many of the same benefits, so, in the spirit of responsible herbal medicine, we recommend its use.

The common mallow does have its advocates, among them Maria Treben in twentieth-century Austria and the journalist and traveler William Cobbett in early nineteenth-century England. Cobbett offers a remarkable encomium of wild mallows, having learned of their value from a French military captive, a follower of Napoleon, in Long Island, New York.

The English farrier, A. Lawson, writing after Cobbett, quotes his own experience of using boiled mallow leaves to treat the badly swollen arm of a nearby farmer and to close a deep wound in a pig that had been gored by a cow's horn. Lawson quotes Cobbett with approval:

*This weed is perhaps amongst the most valuable of plants that ever grew. Its leaves stewed, and applied wet, will cure, and almost instantly cure, any cut or bruise or wound of any sort.... And its operation is in all cases so quick that it can hardly be believed.*

For her part, Treben writes of making up a mallow gargle to treat a man with cancer of the larynx. She used the residue of the mallow mixture, mixed with barley flour, as an overnight poultice for the man's throat. Within two weeks, he was well enough to consider a return to his profession of teaching. The man's medical specialist said of Treben, "This woman deserves a gold medal!"

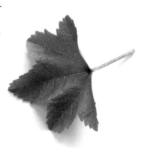

*Now, a person must be almost criminally careless not to make a provision of this herb.... If the use of this weed were generally adopted, the art and mystery of healing wounds, and of curing sprains, swellings and other external maladies, would very quickly be reduced to an unprofitable trade.*
– Cobbett (c1820s)

At an earlier date, Nicholas Culpeper had written movingly of saving his son from "inside plague" by using a mallow liquor [see panel on right]. In the sixteenth century and later, mallow had a reputation as *omnimorbia*, literally a cure-all. This could have been because mallow is laxative, and this was thought to rid the body of all disease.

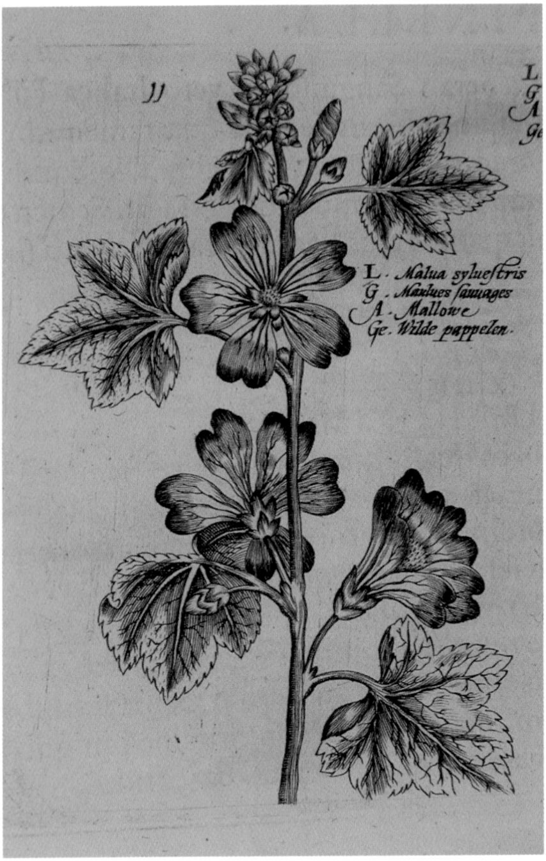
11
L. Malua syluestris
G. Mauues sauuages
A. Mallowe
Ge. Wilde pappelen.

### Use mallow for...

While modern-day mallow users would scarcely claim it as a cure-all, they would also say it doesn't merit official oblivion. Mallow does have solid virtues, and most of these arise from its high mucilage content: common mallow flowers have around 10% mucilage and the leaves 7%. Indeed, all thousand or so members of the *Malva* family worldwide possess this gelatinous substance, including okra and hibiscus.

Mucilage, a word that is cognate with mucus, is extremely soothing to any inflamed part of the body, both outside and within. This includes dry coughs, colds, gastrointestinal upsets, stomach ulcers, and urinary tract infections. As one herbalist notes, when you cannot even swallow water, you can take a mallow tea. Further, it is very safe, in any quantity.

Maria Treben advocates mallow foot and hand baths for treating swellings following bone fractures.

One thing to watch out for in wild-gathering mallow is that its low-growing crinkly leaves tend to accumulate heavy metals from vehicle exhausts and also attract a mallow rust and various insect eggs. So it is a good idea to do your picking well away from busy roads and examine carefully any leaves and flowers you collect.

Mallow from *Hortus Floridus* (1614–16), by Crispijn van de Passe

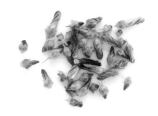

Mallow is sometimes eaten as a soup, though it is rather "gloupy," and the unripe seed heads make a slightly astringent addition to salads. These seed capsules have long been known as "cheeses," but because of the circular shape rather than the taste. The flowers were chewed to relieve toothache.

Always with mallow, though, you come back to its unrivaled soothing benefits. But do remember that large doses can be laxative as well as purgative! Cicero (106–43 BC) angrily reports being accidentally purged by eating a stew of mallow mixed with beet – and he laments that he had already forgone the oysters in an effort to be good.

*You may remember that not long since there was a raging disease called the bloody-flux; the college of physicians not knowing what to make of it, called it the inside plague, for their wits were at Ne plus ultra about it.*

*My son was taken with the same disease, and the excoriation of his bowels was exceeding great; myself being in the country, was sent for up, the only thing I gave him, was Mallows bruised and boiled both in milk and drink, in two days (the blessing of God being upon it) it cured him.*

*And I here, to shew my thankfulness to God, in communicating it to his creatures, leave it to posterity.*
*– Culpeper (1653)*

---

## Harvesting mallow
Pick the leaves before the plant flowers or whenever they are a bright healthy green. They are best used fresh, although they can be dried.

Pick the flowers and flower buds in summer. They can be used fresh or dried by spreading them out on a sheet of paper in a cool airy place. Mallow flowers turn from pinkish purple to blue as they dry. They can be used on their own as a soothing tea, and make a pretty addition to other herbal tea blends.

## Mallow poultice
Chop or chew a fresh mallow leaf and apply to swellings, wounds, and cuts. The poultice can be held in place using a sticking plaster or bandage for as long as it is needed. It reduces inflammation as it soothes and heals, so is good for insect bites, boils, and abscesses.

## Mallow tea
Use a rounded teaspoonful of the **dried or fresh flowers** or a couple of **fresh leaves** per mugful of boiling water. Allow to infuse for about 5 minutes, then strain.

**Dose:** Drink a mugful 3 times a day as needed to soothe the digestion, or coughs and sore throats.

## Mallow salad
Mallow leaves and petals make a mild and pleasant addition to a leafy green salad, and make it warmer and more soothing to the digestion.

**Mallow poultice**
• swellings
• insect bites
• boils & abscesses
• cuts

**Mallow tea**
• indigestion
• IBS
• dry, sore throat
• dry cough
• mild constipation

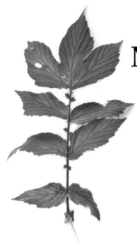

# Meadowsweet *Filipendula ulmaria*

The story of meadowsweet, queen of the meadow, links mead, Cuchulainn, Queen Elizabeth I, and the invention of aspirin.

This is the number one herb for treating stomach acid problems, while also benefiting the joints and urinary system. Meadowsweet is effective for fevers and flu, diarrhea, headaches and pain relief generally. It well earns its name "herbal aspirin."

**Rosaceae**
**Rose family**

**Description:** A perennial of up to 4 or 5 feet tall, with serrated leaves, silvery beneath, and fragrant masses of creamy-white flowers in high summer.

**Habitat:** Marshes, streams, ditches, and moist woodland.

**Distribution:** Widespread in its native Europe, introduced to north-eastern North America.

**Related species:** There are ten species in the genus worldwide.

**Parts used:** Flowering tops; less often, leaves and roots.

A European wild plant, fortunately more common now there is less spraying on field edges and hedgerows, meadowsweet has some delightful country names, including queen or lady of the meadow, maid of the mead, bride-

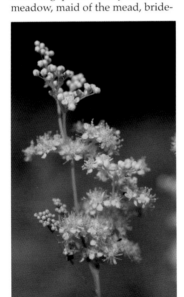

wort, and sweet or new mown hay. But plant historians suggest the origin of the common name is more to do with mead the honey drink than meadows as such. Meadsweet is another old name, and William Turner's herbal (1568) has "medewurte," a term also used by Chaucer two centuries earlier.

The creamy billows of meadowsweet's flowers have indeed been used for centuries as a flavoring for mead, wine, beer, and syrups, and still make a good choice.

Everybody says the smell is full of summer echoes, but some do find it rather overpowering. Matthew is one of these, and says: "I owe a lifelong debt to meadowsweet as this was the very first long word I uttered. At about three years old, according to my mother, when I was saying almost nothing else, out pops this word I'd heard on family walks in the Trent marshes. These days I'm more likely to swear, though, as I get hayfever if I'm too close to the flowers."

In herbal medicine terms, the plant gives much more than it takes. A sacred herb of the Druids, meadowsweet was well known to Celtic communities as a malaria and fever treatment. The legendary hero Cuchulainn was given it to calm his fits of rage and fevers, as recalled in the plant's Gaelic name, "belt of Cuchulainn."

**Use meadowsweet for...**
The flowers and tops yield a beneficial herb tea or tincture that is particularly good for an upset stomach and diarrhea, and the whole plant was a traditional strewing herb of medieval and Tudor times. Charles I's herbalist, John Parkinson, wrote in 1640:

*because both flowers and herbes are of so pleasing a sweete sent, many doe much delight therein, to have it layd in their Chambers, Parlars, &c. and Queene Elizabeth of famous memory, did more desire it then any other sweet herbe to strew her Chambers withall.*

Willow has a longer record of use in pain relief, with Hippocrates, "the father of medicine," in the fifth century BC, using powdered willow bark and leaves to control headache and pain generally. But it was research on meadowsweet that led to chemical breakthroughs in the nineteenth century.

These included the identifying of salicylic acid, and culminated in the synthesis and manufacture of it as aspirin. The drug company

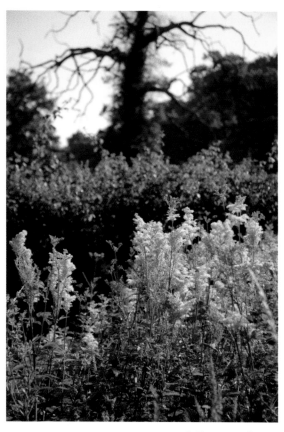

Frothy, creamy flowers, erect reddish stalks, a ditch location: typical meadowsweet in high summer

Bayer patented the name in 1899, basing it on the old Latin name for meadowsweet, *Spiraea*.

We now know that, like willow, meadowsweet contains natural salicylate salts. Aspirin itself is synthesized acetylsalicylic acid, which in concentration the stomach finds burning. This means pure aspirin can cause stomach pain and ulcers, but meadow-

**Cautions:** If you are allergic to aspirin you may have a similar reaction to meadowsweet.

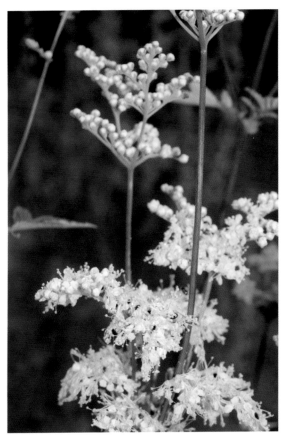

astringency. Instead of damaging the stomach, it soothes upset tummies and is a good remedy for children's diarrhea.

In terms of acid indigestion, reducing the acid levels in the stomach can assist in lowering such levels in the body overall. This might explain why meadowsweet is so effective in treating joint problems associated with acidity.

It has been used to good effect in dispelling uric and oxalic acid, thereby relieving some of the pain of articular rheumatism and gout. A stronger infusion is taken in such cases. Externally, cloths soaked in meadowsweet tea can also be applied to sore joints and bring extra relief; another soothing external use is for mouth ulcers and bleeding gums.

One other area of benefit is in the positive effect of the plant's salicylates for treating cystitis and urethritis, as well as breaking down kidney stones and gravel. The strong capacity of the plant to eliminate toxins and uric acid supports this action.

*... the plant exerts the same effects and is prescribed for the same complaints [as aspirin], but with the bonus of being a natural remedy.*
– Palaiseul (1973)

*... an excellent "herbal aspirin."*
– Cech (2000)

sweet's balanced combination of organic compounds is soothing for heartburn and hyperacidity, as well as ulcers.

This is not to decry aspirin, for like meadowsweet it offers a wonderful combination of pain-relieving and anti-inflammatory benefits. The plant, however, has a broader range of activity, including gentle

Meadowsweet always brings its analgesic and soothing properties to even the more vigorous aspects of its healing range, and as a relaxant it stops spasm and promotes restorative sleep. And even if you are feeling well, if you have the tea to hand, all you have to do is smell it, and you'll feel summer's heat and brightness return.

### Harvesting meadowsweet

Pick **meadowsweet flowers** and **leaves** on a dry sunny day. Spread them on paper or a screen outside for a while to let all the little black beetles escape, then dry indoors. Once dry, crumble or cut into smaller pieces and store in brown paper bags or in jars, in a cool dark place.

### Meadowsweet tea

Use a rounded teaspoonful of the **dried meadowsweet** per mug of **boiling water**, and allow to infuse for 5 minutes. It's best made in a teapot or covered mug to keep the aroma in. Drink a cup before meals if you suffer from acid indigestion or stomach problems, or one to three cups a day for arthritic and rheumatic aches and pains.

### Meadowsweet glycerite

Pick **meadowsweet flowers** on a dry sunny day. Spread them on a cloth outside and let any insects escape, then pack the flowers into a jar large enough to hold them. Make a mix of 60% **vegetable glycerine** with 40% **water** (ie for 10 fl oz, you would use 6 fl oz glycerine and 4 fl oz water), and pour this mixture onto the meadowsweet until the jar is full. Stir to release any trapped air bubbles and top up if necessary.

Put the jar on a sunny windowsill, pushing the flowers back under the liquid every few days if necessary, or employ a plastic 'preserving plunger' used in jam-making to keep it down. It's a good idea to put a saucer under your jar, as sometimes the glycerine will ooze out at the top. After two weeks, strain off the liquid, bottle, and label it.

**Dose:** 1 teaspoonful three times a day for stomach problems. A teaspoonful can also just be taken just when it's needed for heartburn and indigestion, with a second dose after an hour if necessary.

### Meadowsweet electuary

For a particularly irritated digestive tract, mix **slippery elm powder** into your **meadowsweet glycerite** to make a runny paste or electuary.
**Dose:** 1 teaspoonful three times a day as needed.

### Meadowsweet ghee

This is a lovely warming, pain-relieving rub, which goes on smoothly and smells of summer sweetness. To make the ghee, take a packet of **butter** and melt it in a small saucepan. Simmer for about 20 minutes, skim off and discard the foam on top, then slowly pour the clear golden liquid into a clean saucepan leaving behind the whitish residue at the bottom. Put 5 or 6 heads of **meadowsweet flowers** in the ghee and heat gently for about 10 minutes. Strain and pour into jars to set.

**Meadowsweet tea**
- indigestion
- heartburn
- excess stomach acid
- gastritis
- hiatus hernia
- stomach ulcer
- arthritis
- rheumatism

**Meadowsweet glycerite**
- indigestion
- heartburn
- excess stomach acid
- gastritis
- hiatus hernia
- stomach ulcer
- arthritis
- rheumatism

**Meadowsweet electuary**
- heartburn
- diverticulitis
- bowel inflammation

**Meadowsweet ghee**
- muscle aches & pains
- sciatica
- backache
- painful joints
- arthritis

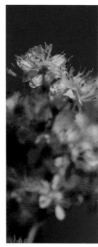

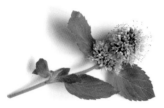

# Mint *Mentha* spp.

**Mint is wonderful for the digestion, as a tea, in food and medicinally. It also relieves nausea, spasms, and gas, and offers the benefits of being both warming and cooling to the body.**

**Lamiaceae (Labiatae) Deadnettle family**

**Description:** Aromatic perennials with dense whorls of lilac flowers.

**Habitat:** Most species prefer stream sides and damp places in woods or grassland.

**Distribution:** Native and naturalized mints are found around the world.

**Species:** Peppermint (*M.* x *piperita*) and field or wild mint (*M. arvensis*) are native and widespread in North America and Europe. Other European species such as water mint (*Mentha aquatica*), pennyroyal (*M. pulegium*), spearmint (*M. spicata*), and apple or round-leaved mint (*M. suaveolens*) are naturalized in North America. They hybridize easily with each other and with garden mints. Any of them can be used, but avoid pennyroyal if you are pregnant.

**Parts used:** Leaves and flowers, harvested in spring and summer.

A hot, hazy, sultry afternoon in high summer, under a high blue sky with scudding white clouds. We are visiting a wet part of the wood behind our house. Water mint and peppermint abound, at their washed-out purple peak, along with the almost identical colors of hemp agrimony and the commoner thistles.

This is an example of collective taking of turns as plants of similar color ripen together. The pale purple flowers are active this week along with attendant pollinators. Butterflies, bees, flies, and smaller insects are pulled to the mints, and red admirals, peacocks, meadow browns, commas, and whites feast on the flowers. Photographing them is another matter, but eventually a meadow brown stays still.

It's one of those days when herbal medicine is at its most pleasant and mellow, with the sweet tang of bruised mint and lazy buzz of insects giving us a feeling we have taken to calling content-mint.

But what do we mean by "mint"? There are at least two dozen different species and hundreds of cultivars, if you add the wild and garden mints together. Moreover, the mints hybridize willingly and produce subtle new forms. As a ninth-century treatise on plants put it, "if one were to enumerate completely all the virtues, varieties and names of mint, one would be able to say how many fish are swimming in the Red Sea…"

We must simplify, and suggest you can use any garden or wild mint. Mints are chemically divided by smell and taste into pepperminty mints and spearminty mints, though there are many variations.

What we usually mean by "mint" is probably peppermint (*M. piperita*), which has flourished in gardens and in the wild since the seventeenth century. It is considered to be a hybrid of watermint and spearmint, but has a stronger proportion of aromatic oils than either. These oils, particularly menthol, account for the greater "mintiness" of peppermint and for its commercial use.

Modern commercial uses of mint build on older and proven herbal applications, but to our mind the focus on taste has all but negated the original herbal virtues.

### Use mint for…

Finding that mint cleaned the breath and settled the digestion, Romans of classical times valued it; they didn't have chocolate, but they did have after-dinner mint! They also brought mint to Britain. Perhaps, indeed, chewing mint leaves is superior, given that our chocolate "mint" doesn't contain any of the herb, and precious little of its oil. It's also moot whether it'd be better for us to clean our teeth on freshly picked mint than use a spurious "mint" toothpaste.

Peppermint's higher levels of aromatic oils come with necessary

*The savor or smell of the water Mint re-joyceth the heart of man, for which cause they use to strew it in chambers and places of recreation, pleasure, and repose, and where feasts and banquets are made.*
– Gerard (1597)

*"Altogether," says Dr Braddon, "the oil of Peppermint forms the best, safest, and most agreeable of known antiseptics."*
– William Thomas Fernie (1897)

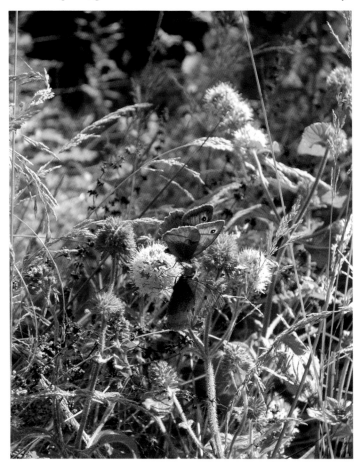

The essence of summer: flowering mint, meadow grasses, sultry sunshine, and feeding butterflies. Norfolk, England in July

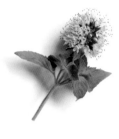

cautions, especially if you use peppermint essential oil. For example, while a mint tea of any species is soothing to the stomach, taking peppermint essential oil internally can lead to stomach spasms; it has been implicated in miscarriages. A drop or two of the essential oil, diluted with a carrier oil and applied to the brow, can relieve a migraine but larger quantities can cause bad headaches.

*The vertues of the wild Mints are more especially to dissolve winde in the stomack, to help the chollick and those that are short-winded, and are an especiall remedy for those that have venerous dreames and pollutions in the night, used both inwardly, and the juyce being applyed outwardly to the testicles or cods.*
– Parkinson (1640)

Using any of the wild mints is considered safe, although pennyroyal should not be taken in pregnancy. Peppermint is the strongest and most cooling mint and is the "official" mint. Mints with more of a spearmint taste are gentler and warmer, and are better for children's fevers, lack of appetite and weak digestive systems.

Medicinally, mint is classified as both cooling and heating, depending on use, species and form taken. This dual energetic pattern, tellingly, is recognized in traditional Chinese, Ayurvedic and western herbal traditions. You can feel the effect when taking mint tea: it warms, then cools the palate and digestion, even the skin; it is stimulating and then soothing.

The heating effect is seen in the way mint is used as a heart tonic, which relieves palpitations, sending blood to the skin's surface, in the form of sweating. Hot mint tea is an excellent recourse for disturbed digestion, relieving spasms and relaxing the stomach walls,

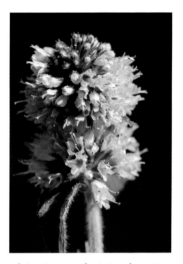

while also anesthetizing them. It is a proven and peerless remedy for such socially embarrassing conditions as bad breath, flatulence, and hiccups; it works for indigestion, bloating, griping, colic, nausea, and vomiting (including morning and travel sickness).

Mint is also antiseptic and mildy antiviral and antifungal. It combats mouth ulcers caused by *Herpes simplex* virus. It is good for coughs, colds, and fever, alone or with elderberry. It also has a traditional use in treating gallstones and for hives, sinusitis and emphysema, earache and toothache, all in addition to its culinary versatility. And, who knows, as Parkinson writes (see left), mint may still be used to reduce "venerous dreames and pollutions in the night," if that is what you want.

**Caution:** Avoid taking pennyroyal if you are pregnant.

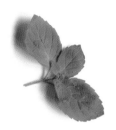

## Mint tea

**Fresh mint** is better than dried to use for tea. Put a couple of sprigs in a teapot and pour in a cupful of **boiling water**. Cover and let infuse for a few minutes before straining and drinking.

But when you do not have fresh mint available, dried is still good. Dry the leaves on a screen outdoors or in a warm cupboard, until they crumble in the fingers. Use a teaspoonful per cup. Dried mint is a very useful addition to other medicinal herb teas, to make them taste better.

## Mint and raspberry water

**Water** can be deliciously and subtly flavored by adding a few sprigs of **mint** and some **raspberries,** and left to stand in a cool place for a couple of hours. Either still or sparkling water can be used. This is a lovely cooling and refreshing summer drink.

If you want a stronger flavor, add a little cool mint tea to the jug.

## Sekanjabin: A Persian oxymel of mint and vinegar

Boil **1 cup of water** with **4 tsp of white sugar**, till the sugar dissolves. Add **1/2 cup of vinegar** (we like to use raspberry vinegar). Simmer for 20 minutes, stirring occasionally.

Remove from heat and add some sprigs of **fresh mint**, which adds its flavor to the oxymel as it cools. Serve diluted in ice-cold water, as you would a cordial. Alternatively, freeze in the form of ice cubes and store for future use.

## Mint in white wine

Put a few sprigs of **mint** and a bottle of **white wine** in a jug, cover with a cloth and leave overnight. Remove the mint. This is a refreshing summer drink that can be served chilled, to keep you cool and improve your digestion.

For a more medicinal apéritif, add a few heads of meadowsweet blossom and a couple of sprigs of mugwort to your wine as well as the mint. This can be done at the same time or added later.

## Mint foot bath

Make a big pot of **mint tea**, strain it and pour it into a foot bath or a basin large enough for your feet. When it is the right temperature, put your feet in the liquid and soak for ten to twenty minutes. Use it hot for tired, achy feet or cold if your feet are really hot and sweaty.

**Mint tea**
- indigestion
- colds and flu
- hot conditions
- flatulence
- nausea
- travel sickness
- headache
- stomach pains

**Sekanjabin**
- hot conditions
- lack of appetite
- weak digestion
- indigestion

**Mint in white wine**
- lack of appetite
- weak digestion
- indigestion

**Mint foot bath**
- tired, achy feet
- hot, sweaty feet

*God's wrath is His vinegar, mercy His honey.*
*These two are the basis of every oxymel.*
*If vinegar overpowers honey, a remedy is spoiled.*
*The people of the earth poured vinegar on Noah;*
*the Ocean of Divine Bounty poured sugar.*
*The Ocean replenished his sugar,*
*and overpowered the vinegar of the whole world.*
*– Rumi (13th-century Persia)*

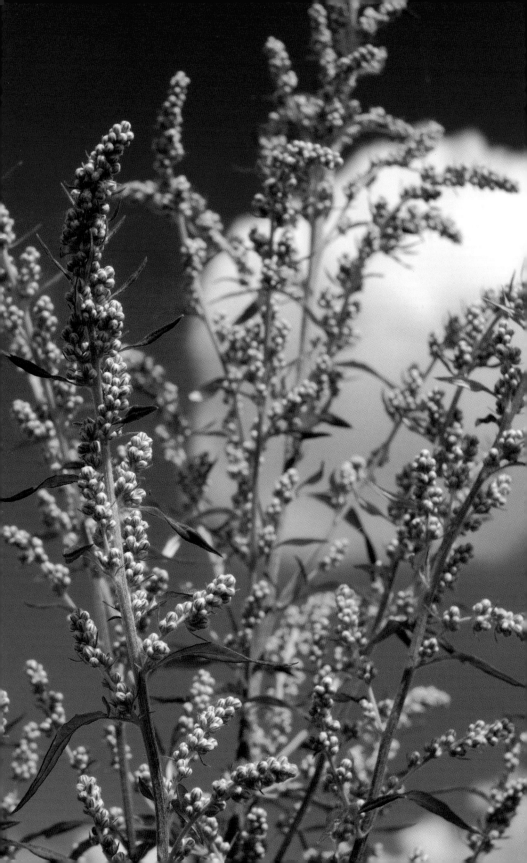

# Mugwort, common wormwood

*Artemisia vulgaris*

**Mugwort is a stately, self-assured perennial, a tall summer presence at up to 6 or more feet high, found in country and town alike. It is, however, far more than a roadside curiosity.**

**It is an ancient herb of healing, magic, and divination throughout the world, a protector of women and travelers, renowned for its value in feminine disorders, and as a strong warming tonic. Mugwort was used in making ale in Europe before hops.**

**Asteraceae (Compositae) Daisy family**

**Description:** A tall, slightly aromatic per-ennial with silvery flower spikes, growing to 6 ft or more. Leaves are pinnate, dark green, and smooth above, silver beneath.

**Habitat:** Waysides, roadsides, waste ground.

**Distribution:** Found across Europe to Asia and North America.

**Related species:** Worldwide, there are hundreds of species of *Artemisia*, including tarragon (*A. dracunculus*), the North American sagebrushes, Chinese mugwort (*A. verlotiorum*) and wormwood (*A. absinthium*). Many of them are used medicinally.

**Parts used:** Flowering tops and leaves.

The first clue to mugwort's significance might be found in its scientific name. *Artemis* was the Greek moon goddess and patron of women, especially at critical phases of their life cycle – at the onset of menstruation, in childbirth and at menopause.

*Vulgaris* can mean "of the people," or, a little more condescendingly, "common" and by extension "abundant." A frequently found herb that is available to assist women everywhere for critical times could hardly have a more apt name than *Artemesia vulgaris*.

Such qualities have been recognized far and wide. Mugwort has been called "the mother of herbs" in several cultures. Ayurvedic practitioners in India use it in treating female reproductive disorders; a related species has the same function in southern Africa, and it has long been known in China for regulating the menses and "calming a restless fetus."

Culpeper placed it under the power of Venus; the Pennsylvania Dutch knew mugwort as *Aldy Fraw*, or "old woman," underlining ancestral wisdom and feminine qualities; and a contemporary western herbalist calls it "the feminine remedy *par excellence*."

A saying from the North of England and Scotland underlines the traditional value of female spring tonics: "If nettles were used in March and muggings [mugwort] in May, many a bra' lass wouldna turn t'clay."

Another dimension to mugwort's popularity is its capacity to influence dreams, a powerful attribute in traditional cultures. A bundle of leaves and flower heads placed under the pillow, or made into a "dream pillow," can calm sleep and protect from nightmares. It might also yield lucid dreams in certain people. In this sense mugwort is shamanistic, underlining its use in divination.

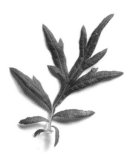

A close-up of mugwort buds and flowers

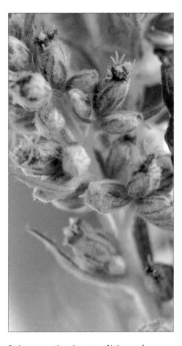

*The leaves and tops of the young shoots and flowers in this plant are all full of virtue, they are aromatic to the taste with a little sharpness. The herb has been famous from the earliest times, and Providence has placed it everywhere about our doors so that reason, and authority, as well as the notice of the senses, point it out for use, but chemistry has banished natural medicines.*
*– Hill (1756)*

It is a continuing tradition of a number of Native American groups to burn bundles of cured and dried sagebrush (*A. tridentata*), a close relative of mugwort, as "smudge sticks." These bundles burn slowly, like an incense stick, producing smoke that is used to cleanse the energy of houses and sacred spaces (see page 109).

Burning a mugwort smudge stick certainly worked in calming the frantic energy when our teenage son had a big boozy party at our home. It also helps shift old, stuck energy – we found ourselves therapeutically clearing out the garden sheds next morning.

## Use mugwort for...

Burning mugwort can dispel midges and other summer biting insects, a quality sometimes suggested as a source of its name (Old Saxon *muggia wort* or midge plant). A case is made too for the Saxon *moughte*, a moth or maggot, referring to mugwort's ability to keep away moths from clothes.

The thirteenth-century Physicians of Myddfai in central Wales knew mugwort as a useful insecticide: "to destroy flies, let the mugwort be put in a place where they are frequent and they will die."

Our own favorite explanation for the name mugwort is its former use as an herbal flavoring for ale. It could have literally been the "mugwort," the measure of a brew, from a time before hops came in during and after the Middle Ages, and the Briton's drink gradually switched from ale to beer. Mugwort, along with yarrow, myrtle, and heather, was a common ingredient in *gruit* or *grut*, a strong herbal ale. This is currently enjoying something of a revival in the modern microbrewery movement.

An infusion of mugwort in cold drinks, whether beer or fruit in origin, adds a sharp summer tang and aromatic smell that you can enjoy in safety. These make for a more homely and less risky prospect than absinthe, the liqueur derived from the closely related wormwood (*A. absinthium*). As the world knows, this was the tipple of the *fin de siècle* French literary and art world. Containing a toxic essential oil that mugwort lacks, absinthe could be fatally addictive. It was banned in Europe for most of the twentieth century.

Mugwort, it will be clear by now, has had something of a dangerous past, at the hazy margin of sacred and secular culture – indeed, from a time when there was no distinction made between the two.

American herbalist Maida Silverman believes that "Folklore and superstition are bound up with the Mugwort plant to an extent hardly matched by any other herb." She instances as the oldest superstition the first-century AD Roman naturalist Pliny, who recommended that travelers carry mugwort as an amulet for psychic protection. This belief lasted through and beyond the Middle Ages, only to be roundly condemned by the "rational" herbalists like Gerard (1597) and Parkinson (1640).

Mugwort was a key Anglo-Saxon sacred herb: the *Leech Book of Bald* from tenth-century Wessex extols it as "eldest of worts / Thou has might for three / And against thirty." Again the great age and protective power of mugwort are emphasized.

In medieval times mugwort passed from the patronage of the pagan Artemis to the Christian care of St John the Baptist, who was said to have carried it into the wilderness to ward off evil. From this came "St John's girdle" and the wearing of a mugwort garland on St John's day, June 24th, while dancing around the traditional fire. Throwing the garland into the fire would ensure protection for the following year, another pagan survival that so annoyed John Parkinson. He would be aghast to learn that a mugwort ceremony still marks midsummer in the Isle of Man (see box on page 108).

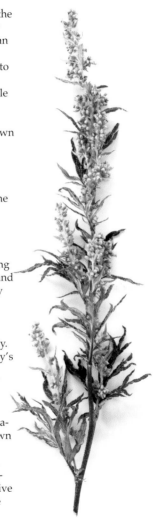

Wider afield, mugwort was known to Chinese medicine as a house protector and in the practice of moxibustion. This is an integral part of acupuncture, and many readers will have experienced the cone of dried mugwort leaves, moxa, being placed on the skin and burnt to stimulate an acupuncture point. The particular application of moxa is for treating abdominal pain from the cold, and it is mugwort's warming quality that makes it effective.

One other aspect of mugwort and fire can be mentioned briefly. Other names for the plant, gypsy's tobacco and muggar, record its persistent use as a smoking leaf inside strips of newspaper.

Burnt or not, mugwort has valuable warming qualities. It is known herbally as an aromatic bitter, which warms the digestion and stimulates a sluggish liver. It encourages the secretion of digestive juices and its oils help eliminate gas and griping.

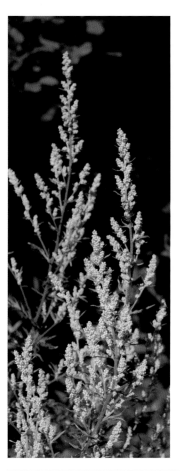

*On a hot summer day, when the noxious fumes and stagnant air in the city seem even more oppressive than usual, it really is a "comfort" to crush a few leaves of the plant in one's hand and inhale the clean, pungent aroma. Mugwort lives up to its reputation and certainly has the power to revive the spirits and refresh the senses.*
*– Silverman (1997)*

Herbalists value mugwort as a general calmer of the nervous system, helping to relieve stress and nervous tension. Mugwort pillows can help soothe disturbed sleep as well as promote dreaming. In general the plant has an uplifting effect on mood and is valuable in treating forms of mild depression linked with digestive weakness.

Taken as a tincture, mugwort can help in normalizing menstrual flow, and is particularly useful for bringing on delayed or suppressed periods where they have been absent for some time. It is a good herb for young women at puberty, helping to establish a regular cycle. Because it stimulates the uterus, it is not normally used in western herbalism during pregnancy, though in China it is an accepted treatment in preventing miscarriage.

Mugwort has some antimalarial activity, though much milder than Sweet Annie (*Artemisia annua*). It is also effective against threadworms and roundworms, like its stronger relative wormwood, and is an effective wash for treating fungal infections.

**Manx mugwort magic**
Mugwort is the symbolic plant of the Isle of Man and sprigs of it are worn on Manx national day, July 5th. This is St John's day in the old Julian calendar (it has been June 24th in England and Scotland since 1752, but the old date is kept on Man). On St John's eve mugwort would be gathered and made into wreaths to be worn by cattle and men alike. Hedge and gorse fires were lit and cattle forced through while men and boys jumped over the flames. This combination of mugwort and fire would protect beast and people from evil spirits for the coming year. The next day was then safe for the many civic ceremonies of Midsummer Court, including the promulgation of laws from Tynwald Hill.
As an invited guest, even Queen Elizabeth II on her visit to Man in 2003 duly wore her spray of mugwort or *bollan bane* (white herb), as it is known locally.

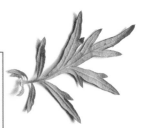

The underside of a mugwort leaf is covered with silvery, downy hairs.

## Harvesting mugwort

Pick mugwort in summer, collecting the flower spikes when they are flowering or just before the flowers open when the buds are still silvery. The leaves can be collected too.

## Mugwort tincture

Because mugwort becomes more aromatic as it dries, the tincture is best made with **dried mugwort**, although you can use fresh. Fill a jar with mugwort, then top up with **vodka**, shaking it to remove air bubbles. Put the jar in a cool dark place for 2 to 4 weeks, then strain and bottle.

**Dose:** Half a teaspoonful, three times a day.

## Mugwort punch

Pour **a cupful of red wine** into a saucepan.
Add **a stick of cinnamon**, **5 cloves**, and **a handful of mugwort tops**. Bring to a boil, then turn down the heat and simmer gently with a lid on for half an hour.
Strain out the herbs and spices. Sweeten with **honey**. It can be taken hot or cold before a meal to stimulate appetite and digestion. Either drink it fresh or keep in a bottle to mature for several weeks.

## Mugwort pillow

Pick **mugwort flowers and leaves** and dry them. Make a small bag for the pillow out of **cloth**, leaving one end open – any size you like, but 8" x 10" works well. Fill the bag loosely with the dried mugwort so that the finished pillow will be about 1" thick, then stitch up the open end. Place this under your regular pillow. Smaller cloth bags of mugwort can be stored among clothing to discourage clothes moths.

## Mugwort smudge stick

Pick the silvery top 8" or so of **mugwort** when the flowers are in bud or first open. Leave them in a cool airy place to dry for a few days. Before they dry completely, and while they are still flexible, make small bundles up to about 1" thick, with the stem ends together. Starting at the stem end, wind a piece of **cotton thread** in a spiral around the bundle to the end and then back again, tying off securely. Leave the bundles to dry completely.

To use, hold the smudge stick by the stem end and light the other end with a match. You may need to blow on it at first to keep it burning. Wave the stick around with a circular motion as you move through a room or around a person – the movement helps keep the stick burning as well as spreading the smoke through the air.

**Mugwort tincture**
- irregular periods
- suppressed periods
- gas and griping
- stress and anxiety

**Mugwort punch**
- poor appetite
- sluggish digestion
- gas and griping
- stress and anxiety

**Mugwort pillow**
- protection from bad dreams
- promotes lucid dreams
- stress and anxiety

**Smudge stick**
- clears negative and old stuck energy
- calms and protects
- warms and dries

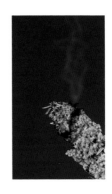

**Scrophulariaceae**
**Figwort family**

**Description:** Biennial plants, growing in their first year as a rosette of downy leaves, and sending up a tall spike with yellow flowers in their second summer.

**Habitat:** Sides of fields, roadsides, dry ground.

**Species used:** Great mullein is the species generally discussed in herbals, but any of the tall, yellow-flowered mulleins can be used, as can white mullein (*Verbascum album*).

**Distribution:** Great mullein (*V. thapsus*) is native to Europe, northern Africa, and Asia, and naturalized in parts of North America, Africa, and Australia.

**Related species:** There are about 300 species of *Verbascum* worldwide.

**Parts used:** Leaves and flowers, sometimes the root.

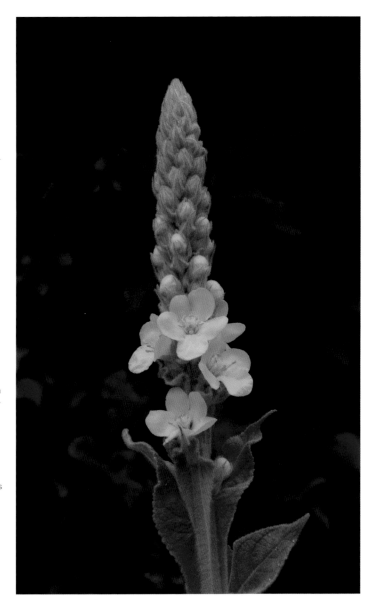

# Mullein *Verbascum* spp.

**Mullein is unmistakable when it is in flower, with its spires of yellow flowers on a spike reaching six feet tall. It likes disturbed ground and dry soil, often growing on roadsides.**

**The flowers, infused in oil, are a remedy for earache and other nerve pain. The leaves and flowers taken as a tea relieve dry irritable coughs. Mullein, so supple and strong itself, has an affinity for the spine and helps in setting bones.**

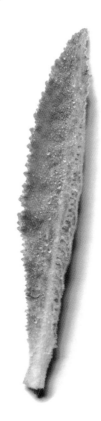

Mullein has a long history of use in Europe, and has been attributed magical powers in several mythologies. Almost three thousand years ago, according to Homer, Odysseus used the root of moly, which was probably the white mullein, as a protection against the enchantments of Circe. Odysseus was lucky to have the help of Hermes, for, in Homer's words, "it was an awkward plant to dig up, at any rate for a mere man. But the gods, after all, can do anything."

There are records of the long stalk of mullein being dipped in tallow and used as a taper by Roman legionaries and in medieval funerals. It also has a reputed association with witches' covens, recalled in the common name hag's taper.

Mullein leaves have made a natural toilet paper, diapers, food wrappers, and soothing insoles for shoes – all possible emergency uses today. Despite their softness, however, mullein leaves can be irritating when dry because of all their little hairs. It is this attribute that gave the plant the name of Quaker rouge, as Quaker girls were said to redden their cheeks by rubbing the leaves on them.

A cure for hoarseness, with mullein and fennel in equal parts, cooked in wine, goes back to Hildegard of Bingen in the 1100s.

John Parkinson (1640) recommends a decoction of the leaves with sage, marjoram, and chamomile (applied externally) for cramps. He mentions that country men gave a broth of mullein to cattle that had coughs and used a poultice of the leaves for horses' hooves injured in shoeing.

A Victorian doctor, Dr Quinlan, publicized a traditional Irish TB treatment in which one handful of fresh mullein leaves was boiled with two pints of milk, strained and sweetened with honey; the mix was to be drunk twice a day.

*Mullein is an herb for the lungs and throat and can be consumed in any rational quantity needed, being basically free of toxicity.*
*– Moore (1979)*

### Use mullein for...

Mullein's soft fuzzy leaves give a hint of its soothing qualities for internal use. Its particular affinity is for the respiratory system, but it also calms and strengthens the nerves, digestion, and urinary system. It is good for swollen glands, and helps relieve pain in general.

Think of mullein tea for easing throat and chest problems, especially dry and irritable coughs. It can quickly soothe an irritating tickle at the back of the throat.

Mullein flower oil is the best natural remedy for earache. Our son's ear infections when he was little were always quickly relieved

*Mullein is the only herb known to man that has remarkable narcotic properties without being poisonous and harmful.*
*– Dr Christopher (1976)*

(except for once when the oil was old and had lost its potency). The oil can be used externally for any kind of swelling and irritation.

Following up on ancient precedent, a useful remedy to ease the foot pain of plantar fasciitis is to put a fresh mullein leaf in your shoe, replacing with a new one when the first one has dried out.

Mullein poultices for external use are excellent to draw out splinters and boils, but, like the tea, also work at deeper bodily levels for backaches, lymphatic swellings, and even broken bones. The poultices are effective in soothing swollen glands and for mumps.

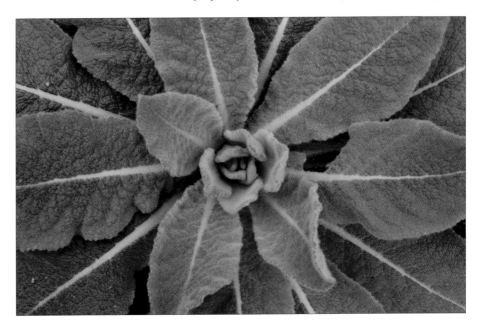

### Harvesting mullein

The leaves are best picked before the plant sends up its flower spike. Dry the leaves whole and then crumble them for storage.

The flowers are quite soft, so pick them carefully to avoid bruising. Spread in a single layer on a sheet of paper or a mesh screen to dry.

### Mullein tea

The leaves can be used on their own, or you can add flowers. To make the tea, use a good rounded tablespoonful of the **dried herb**, slightly more of the fresh, according to taste. Pour a mugful of **boiling water** over it, cover and steep for 15 minutes. Strain through muslin or a fine sieve to remove any loose leaf hairs if you are using the dried leaf. Drink freely for dry coughs or any irritation of throat and chest.

### Mullein flower oil

Pick the **flowers** on a dry sunny day, and lay them on a sheet of paper to dry a little overnight. Put them in a small jar and pour enough **extra virgin olive oil** over them to cover the flowers completely. Close the jar with a piece of cloth held on with a rubber band rather than using a lid – this allows any moisture to escape.

Put the jar on a sunny windowsill for two weeks, stirring every day to keep the flowers submerged in the oil. This is important, as the flowers will tend to float and may go moldy if left exposed.

When the flowers have faded and become quite transparent, the oil is ready to be strained and bottled. Pour through a fine sieve into another jar. There will probably be a layer of water at the bottom of the jar, so the oil needs to be poured slowly and carefully into a third jar, leaving the watery layer behind. Store in a cool dark place for up to a year.

For earache, put 1 to 3 drops of oil in the affected ear as needed for pain.

### Mullein poultice

To make a poultice, lay a few **mullein leaves** in a dish (for a splinter you'll only need part of a leaf) and pour a little **boiling water** on them to soften them. Leave until they are cool enough to handle, then place them on the affected part. The poultice can be held on with a bandage, and you can keep it warm by holding a hot water bottle against it.

This is an excellent treatment for removing splinters, to draw boils, to soothe an aching back, and for any lymphatic swellings. It can also be used to help heal broken bones, such as ribs or toes, that cannot be set.

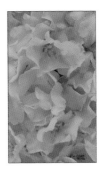

**Mullein tea**
- dry irritable coughs
- bronchitis
- laryngitis
- pleurisy
- swollen glands

**Mullein flower oil**
- earache
- nerve pain
- hemorrhoids & piles
- chest rub
- chilblains

**Tip:** Don't use a bottle with a pipette top for long-term storage of mullein oil. We have found that volatile oils from the mullein destroy the rubber bulb after a while, and the oil loses its potency.

**Mullein poultice**
- splinters
- boils
- backache
- mumps
- swollen glands
- broken bones

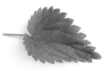

# Nettle, stinging nettle *Urtica dioica*

**Urticaceae**
**Nettle family**

**Description:** A wind-pollinated perennial with dark green, hairy, stinging leaves and stems, and tough, tangled yellow roots.

**Habitat:** Woods, river banks, farms, roadsides, field edges, waste ground, and wherever the nitrogen content of the soil is high.

**Distribution:** Native across North America, Asia and Europe, found in most of the temperate world.

**Related species:** The dwarf or small nettle (*U. urens*), an annual, is similar in use and appearance; it is the species used in homeopathy.

**Parts used:** Leaves, tops, seeds, rhizomes, and roots.

Nettles are one of the most useful of plants, despite their protective sting. The young tops are delicious and nutritious, a natural vitamin and mineral supplement. Medicinally, the leaves, seeds, and roots are used to treat a wide range of conditions including anemia, arthritis, asthma, burns, eczema, infections, inflammations, kidney stones, prostate enlargement, rheumatism, and urinary problems.

Nettles can also be used to make rope, nets, a linen-like cloth and paper, a dye, insect repellant, and green manure.

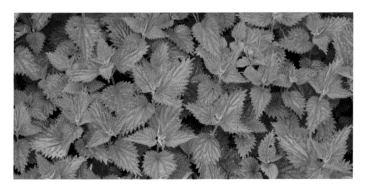

Stinging nettles are one of the best plants for human health, both as food and medicine. They are a complete, ready-packaged natural vitamin and mineral supplement, grow everywhere and are free – an ultimate herbal medicine.

Nettle was the Anglo-Saxon sacred herb, *wergulu*, and in medieval times nettle beer was drunk for rheumatism. Nettle tops helped milk to sour, as a rennet substitute in cheese-making. Nettle leaves brought fruit to ripening, and were used to pack plums; the whole plant is still useful as an excellent compost or green manure.

Nettle's high vitamin C content made it a valuable spring tonic for our ancestors after a winter of living on grain and salted meat, with hardly any green vegetables. Nettle soup and porridge were popular spring tonic purifiers, but a pasta or pesto from the leaves is a worthily nutritious modern alternative. We find all but the youngest shoots rather fibrous, and prefer a purée, as in a nettle form of the Indian dish *sag paneer*.

Nettle soup is described by one modern writer as "Springtime herbalism at one of its finest moments." This soup is the Scottish *kail*. Tibetans believe that their sage and poet Milarepa (AD 1052–1135) lived solely on nettle soup for many years, until he himself turned green: a literal green man.

### Use nettle for…

Modern lifestyles need the kind of nutrition that nettle can offer. It is now known that the mineral content of intensively farmed foods has decreased dramatically over the past half-century, so even people eating a healthy diet may be mineral-deficient. Mineral deficiency contributes to a wide range of chronic health problems, including diabetes and cardiac disease, so nettles can improve diverse conditions purely through their mineral content.

Nettles have an antihistamine effect, valuable for treating hayfever and other allergies. They can help reduce the severity of asthma attacks. For treating hayfever, they combine well with elderflower.

Nettles enhance natural immunity, helping protect us from infections. Nettle tea drunk often at the start of a feverish illness is beneficial. It can be combined with elderflower, lime blossom, yarrow, or mint.

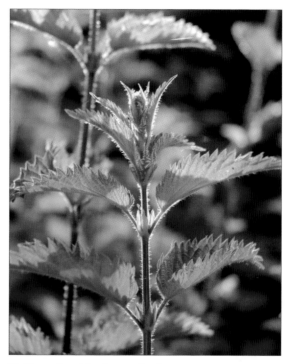

Nettles reduce blood sugar levels and stimulate the circulation, which supports treatment of diabetes. They also dilate the peripheral blood vessels and promote elimination of urine, which helps lower high blood pressure.

Taking nettles has an amphoteric effect on breast milk production, meaning that mothers make more milk if the flow is scanty or less if the flow is excessive.

Nettles have long been considered a blood tonic and are a wonderful treatment for anemia, as they are

The sting from nettles comes from the hairs, which are like tiny glass syringes that inject a stinging acid fluid

*It is more appropriate that nature has given this plant the protection of [a] stinging exterior. Without it, we should probably never have the opportunity to benefit from its healing power. Animals, with their instinctive knowledge of what is good for them, would not leave us even one leaf.*
– Dr Vogel (1989)

Stinging nettle and one of the insects using it as a food plant, the peacock butterfly and larva, by Maria Merian, 1717

high in both iron and chlorophyll. The iron in nettles is very easily absorbed and assimilated.

The root is a leading herbal treatment for enlarged prostate, taken on its own as a tincture or with saw palmetto (*Serenoa repens*).

Stinging nettles help clear the blood of urates and toxins, partly through stimulating the kidneys. Nettle tops make a tea for treating gout and arthritis. Another old arthritis remedy is to whip the

affected joints with fresh nettles (*Urtica urens* has a stronger effect than *U. dioica*). This creates a temporary nettle rash but alleviates pain and stiffness.

If you think this is odd behavior, consider sado-botany, in which sexual partners beat each other with nettles for stimulation and pain/pleasure. The Romans and Greeks of old took nettle seed as an aphrodisiac.

What cooks will tell you is that two minutes of boiling nettle leaves will neutralize both the silica "syringes" of the stinging cells and the histamine or formic acid-like fluid that is so painful.

But if you are brave you can try munching raw leaves. Pinch the top shoot on a young nettle, roll into a tight ball and eat – delicious. This, incidentally, is the technique used in the world nettle-eating championship, held annually in Dorset (eat all the nettles you can in an hour, washed down by beer – the event is sponsored by a pub).

Sir John Harington (1607) had just the remedy for these competitors:

*Tho Nettles ftinke, yet make they recompence,/ If your belly by the Collicke paine endures,/ Againft the Collicke Nettle-feed and hony/ Is Phyfick: better none is had for money./ It breedeth fleepe, ftaies vomits, fleams* [blood-letting instruments] *doth foften,/ It helpes him of the Gowte that eates it often.*

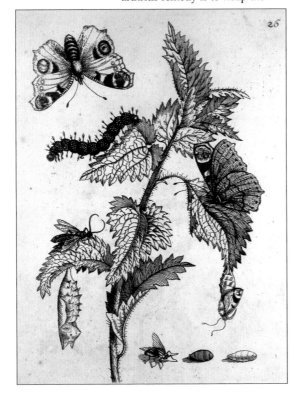

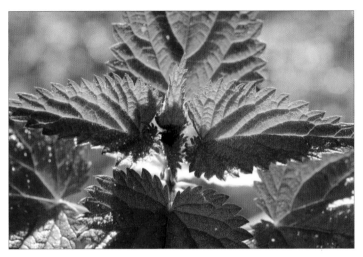

## Harvesting nettle tops

Nettle tops are best in the spring, but if the nettles are repeatedly cut back they will send up fresh shoots, which can be harvested through summer and into autumn. Harvest the top 6", wearing rubber gloves to pick them, or use a pair of scissors to cut and lift them into a bag or basket.

Rinse them if they need it. Young spring nettles can be frozen for use later in the year. Blanch them in boiling water for two minutes, then drain and cool. Chop up or leave whole, and store in freezer bags.

## Nettle tea

Use a couple of fresh **nettle tops** in a teapot per cup of **boiling water**, and allow to infuse for 15 to 20 minutes. This tastes so much better than any nettle tea you can buy. Drink as often as you like. Can also be used as a hair rinse and massaged into the scalp to promote hair growth.

## Nettle juice powder

Juice fresh **nettle tops**, then mix the juice with enough nettle leaf powder (made by reducing **dried nettle tops** in a coffee grinder, then putting the powder through a sieve) to the thickness of double cream. Spread on fruit leather trays in a dehydrator or on non-stick baking trays in a warm oven until dry. Crumble and store in airtight jars.

**Dose:** Half to one teaspoonful daily.

**NETTLE TOPS**
**Tea**
• spring tonic
• anemia
• bleeding
• diarrhea
• gout
• fluid retention
• low blood pressure
• high blood pressure
• coughs
• allergies
• regulates breast milk production
• skin problems
• high blood sugar
**Externally**
• cuts and wounds
• hair tonic

**Juice powder**
• spring tonic
• anemia
• gout
• fluid retention
• low blood pressure
• high blood pressure
• allergies
• regulates breast milk production
• skin problems
• high blood sugar

**NETTLE TOPS**
**Tincture**
- stops bleeding
- promotes urine flow
- burns
- skin problems

**Nettle soup**
- spring tonic
- anemia

### Nettle top decocted tincture

By boiling nettles, you get the minerals that are not extracted well by alcohol. Chop up your **nettle tops**, and divide into two even batches. Put one half in a blender with enough 40% **vodka** to blend, and liquidize. Put the other half in a saucepan with just enough **water** to cover, bring to a boil and simmer for 15 minutes. Allow to cool.

Strain and measure both liquids, then combine, making sure the volume of alcohol is equal to or greater than the volume of water. (If your water volume is greater, return it to the saucepan and simmer down until it is a little less.) Bottle and label.

**Dose:** 1 teaspoonful three times a day. For burns, hold the burn under cold running water for a few minutes first if possible, then wet a cotton wool ball with the tincture and hold it on the burn until the pain eases.

### Nettle soup

Sauté 1 or 2 chopped **onions** in a little **ghee, butter, or olive oil** until the onions are lightly browned. Add about a litre of **water or vegetable stock,** and several handfuls of **fresh nettle tops**. Simmer gently for 10 or 15 minutes, then purée with a hand blender and serve. You can add nutmeg, pepper, or other spices to taste. Then add cream, potatoes, sorrel, or whatever you like – the possible variations are endless.

*Nettle flowers are soon followed by the seeds*

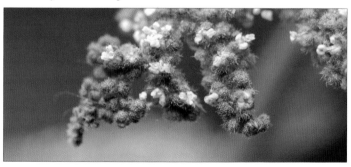

**NETTLE SEED**
**Electuary**
- kidney support
- coughs
- yin tonic (TCM)
- aphrodisiac
- convalescence

### Nettle seed electuary

Cut nettle tops when the **seed** is almost ripe and lay them outdoors on brown paper. This allows any small insects that live on them the time to escape. When dry, strip the seeds off the stems. Grind the seeds in a coffee grinder and mix the powder into a paste with **runny honey**. Store in wide-mouthed jars.

**Dose:** 1 or 2 teaspoonfuls daily.

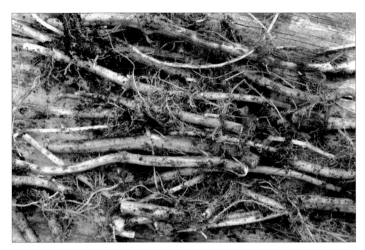

### Harvesting nettle roots

Nettle roots can be dug up whenever they are needed, but are probably at their best in the fall. You will need a stout digging fork and a pair of close-fitting gloves. The yellow roots are tenacious and tangled.

Wash them thoroughly and cut into pieces an inch or two long. To dry, spread them on a cake rack or a screen; put in a warm dry place until brittle.

### Nettle root decoction

Simmer a handful of dried or fresh **nettle root** in a litre of **water** for 20 minutes, then strain.

**Dose:** Drink a cupful two or three times daily, storing the rest in the fridge until you need it and then reheating.

### Nettle root decocted tincture

Put fresh or dried **nettle roots** in a saucepan with enough **water** to cover them, and simmer for 20 minutes. When cool, pour off and measure the liquid, but keep the roots. Add an equal amount of 40% **vodka** to the liquid and pour it in a large jar or jars with the roots. Add a few handfuls of fresh chopped roots. Put the jars in a cupboard and leave for 3 to 4 weeks, shaking occasionally. Strain off and bottle the liquid.

**Dose:** 1 teaspoonful daily to maintain prostate health, or three times daily for more acute problems.

**NETTLE ROOT**
**Decoction**
• prostate enlargement
• infections
• inflammation
• bacterial and fungal infections

**Decocted tincture**
• prostate enlargement
• infections
• inflammation
• bacterial and fungal infections

**Caution:** Do not take nettle root during pregnancy.

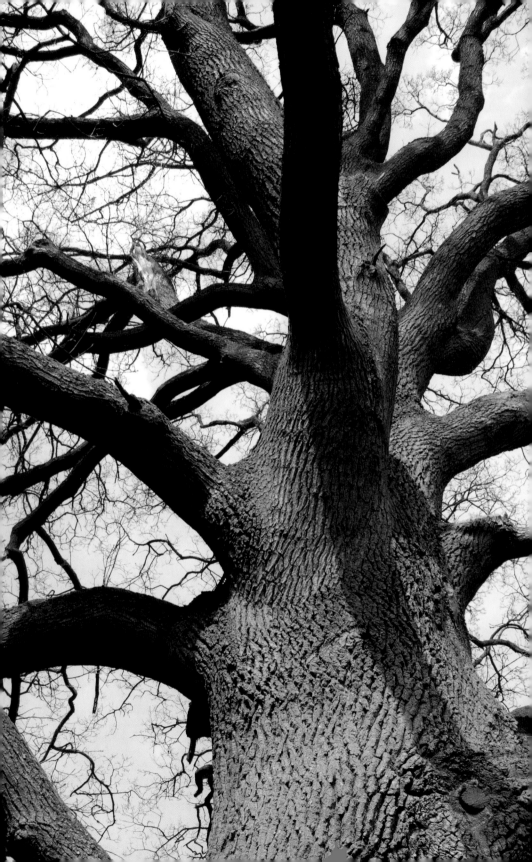

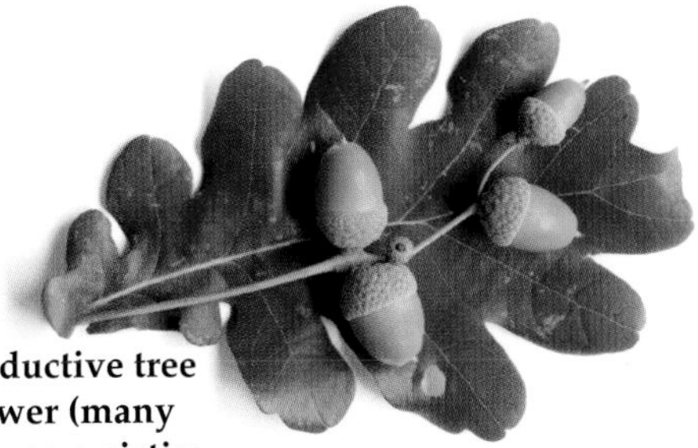

# Oak  *Quercus robur, Q. petraea, Q. alba*

**Oak has been a sacred and an economically productive tree for millennia, the symbol of Britain's secure power (many other countries rightly claim it too). But it has been a victim of its own success, with most of its old forests now gone.**

**In terms of herbal medicine it still has uses, mainly of the bark, leaves, and acorns rather than the galls used in earlier times. Oak is also one of Dr Bach's original flower essences, so its subtle authority lives on.**

We have chosen the picture on the left from among many we've taken of oak in order to convey something of the massive presence and protecting influence of this most stalwart of trees.

There is insufficient space to relate the myths, sacred and secular, the uses, and the central role of oak in the British consciousness. Geoffrey Grigson points out that it has been too necessary and familiar a tree to allow any other general names than its own: oak it is.

Suffice it to say that oak's timber built houses, cathedrals, and ships, made furniture, barrels, and pews; its bark tanned leather for shoes and saddles, and provided dyes; its acorns fed pigs and was a famine food or coffee substitute; its galls (oak apples) gave ink; its wood supplied fuel and charcoal; the tree was a space for mistletoe, ivy, and ferns; it sheltered insects, birds, animals – and outlaws (Robin Hood) and kings (Charles II).

There was once a saying that oak was so important that a person came in contact with it every day of their life, from newborn's cradle to old man's coffin. Such a universal and steadying presence has been lost in modern times, but the tree still offers uses for an enthusiast of herbal medicine.

## Use oak for…

The **bark** is the "official" botanical drug, used as an astringent. The *British Herbal Pharmacopoeia* specifies dried bark from younger stems and branches of *Quercus robur*, though herbalists in practice find that other oak species can be used interchangeably and that acorns, leaves, and oak apples, also rich in tannins, have equivalent benefits (nobody uses oak root!).

Tannins were first isolated chemically from oak bark, and it is thought that "tannin" came from a Celtic term for oak. Oak, tannins, and leather tanning have always been synonymous.

**Fagaceae**
**Beech family**

**Description:** A well-loved tree, which grows to 130 feet tall and can live for a thousand years. The lobed leaves are mainly deciduous, and the flowers are catkins borne in spring. Acorns in little cups are diagnostic for all oaks.

**Habitat:** Forests, woods, parkland.

**Distribution:** The English or pedunculate oak (*Quercus robur*) is native to most of Europe, and is found naturalized in parts of North America. The sessile or Durmast oak (*Q. petraea*) is a European species. White oak (*Q. alba*) is found across eastern North America.

**Species:** White oak (*Q. alba*) is the main North American species used medicinally. The American oaks with rounded leaves generally have edible acorns, while the oaks with pointy leaves have acorns that are high in tannin and very bitter.

**Parts used:** Bark, leaves, acorns, galls.

Astringents are the body's tighteners and driers, being effective in binding and toning tissue and reducing excess discharges. The conditions treated by astringent herbs include diarrhea, dysentery, eye, mouth, and throat inflammations, disturbed mucous membranes of the digestive tract, and bleeding, burns, and sores.

Astringents are also anti-microbial and antiseptic, helping to create a barrier against infection. Herbalist David Hoffmann explains this by saying "astringents produce a kind of temporary leather coat on the surface of tissue."

Oak bark is most often taken as a decoction, small strips of bark from young branches being boiled in water for 10–15 minutes and drunk. It is strong and bitter from the 15% to 20% of tannins it contains, and is the primary treatment for acute diarrhea, taken in small but plentiful doses. If self-medication for diarrhea is not successful after three or four days, the usual advice is to consult a professional.

The same preparation is good as a mouthwash for gargling in sore throats, tonsillitis, and laryngitis, as a douche for leucorrhea, and as an enema for hemorrhoids.

In Germany the "official" uses for oak bark decoction include inflammation of gums and throat, sweating of the feet, chilblains, and anal fissures (the last three in a bath at room temperature). The dried young bark is also powdered in a grinder as a tooth powder, as in our recipe on the next page.

The **leaves** of oak in spring have been used hot as a tea to relieve diarrhea, and after cooling as a soothing compress for sore eyes. Culpeper writes that the distilled water of oak leaves is "one of the best remedies I know of for the whites [leucorrhea] in women." In the field, chewing the leaves and applying them to bites, open wounds, or ulcers eases inflammation and promotes healing.

**Acorns** are the signature of oaks worldwide, and well chosen as a symbol for Britain's National Trust. While enjoyed raw by pigs and squirrels, humans find acorns palatable only when cooked after repeated boiling and renewing of the water, the tannins being gradually leached out. Acorns were a famine food for the Anglo-Saxons, but some North American oaks have more palatable acorns, and Native Americans living in forested areas had acorn flour as a staple part of their diet.

During the First World War an ersatz coffee was made in Germany from roasted and ground acorns. The drink is still available today. It is tasty, good for those with poor digestion and has little caffeine.

Acorns were once an herbal specific for alcoholism, a use reflected in a modern homeopathic remedy formulated to control craving.

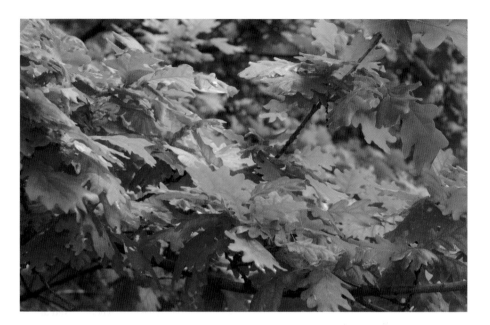

### Oak twig toothbrush

Oak twigs can be used as a natural toothbrush with built-in antiseptic and anti-inflammatory benefits. Simply pick a small twig and chew the end to fray it, then use this to massage your gums and clean your teeth.

### Harvesting oak bark

Select young branches up to about an inch in diameter, and use a sharp knife to remove small strips of bark, cutting along the length of the branch. The bark is thicker than you might expect, brown on the outside but white underneath. Dry the bark strips in a warm place.

### Tooth powder

Break up the dried oak bark into small bits and grind finely in a coffee grinder. Sieve to remove larger pieces. The fennel seed in the recipe can also be ground in this way.

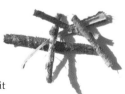

Mix 3 parts **oak bark powder** with 1 part **cinnamon powder**, 1 part **fennel seed powder** and 1 part **bicarbonate of soda**, or to suit your own taste.
Store in a small jar, and use to brush your teeth every day.

**Oak twig tooth-brush**
• gum problems

**Tooth powder**
• gum disease
• weak gums
• bleeding gums
• mouth ulcers

# Pellitory of the wall

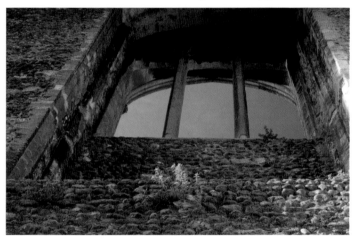

*Parietaria judaica* syn. *P. diffusa, P. officinalis*

**Urticaceae
Nettle family**

**Description:** A red-stemmed perennial with tiny white flowers, growing mainly on walls, to about 2 feet high. Forms dense patches locally.

**Habitat:** Walls, stony places, hedgebanks, and gardens.

**Distribution:** Native to Europe and north Africa, introduced to North America and Australia.

**Related species:** Pennsylvania pellitory (*P. pensylvanica*) is native to North America.

**Parts used:** Above-ground parts.

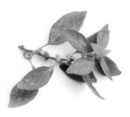

*The dried herbe Paritary made up with hony into an Electuarie, or the juice of the herbe, or the decoction thereof made up with Sugar or Hony, is a singular remedy for any old continuall or dry cough, the shortnesse of breath and wheezings in the throate.
– Parkinson (1640)*

This little and overlooked wild plant is a noted tonic for the kidneys and bladder. It is soothing and increases the flow of urine, while also reducing inflammation and helping dissolve kidney stones. Herbalists use the tea for a range of urinary problems.

Pellitory, named from the Latin *paries* or house wall, was once given a variety of "virtues" or uses, but herbalists today regard it as a specialized urinary tract herb. It is an excellent gentle tonic for cystitis, nephritis, pyelitis, kidney stones, renal colic, and urinary problems linked with prostate enlargement. It will relieve edema and urine retention, and is soothing as well as urine-producing.

In the seventeenth century, John Parkinson and Nicholas Culpeper wrote of using pellitory internally for coughs and uterine pain, and externally for skin problems, burns, and hot conditions. Parkinson said the juice put in the ears "eases the noise and hummings in them" and that the herb "applied to the fundament" opens piles and soothes their pain.

Culpeper had such faith in a syrup made of pellitory juice and honey that he promised free treatment to anyone who took a teaspoonful daily or even just once a week and still got dropsy (edema or fluid retention).

This was a popular remedy at the time. We came across it again in a Norfolk gentleman's notebook:

*For a Dropsie*
*Given mee 18th Novem: 1664 by Mr*
*Sheepeside*
*Take ye juice of Pellitorie of ye wall &*
*boyle it up to a syruppe with honey*
*& so keepe it in a Glasse. Take one*
*spoonefull of this every Morninge.*

Our own preference is to make an infusion as a tea, but a pellitory syrup or even the ale tincture that was once current would be equally effective today.

Pellitory is used in Europe to treat *Herpes zoster* infections, and has possible wider applications in combating viral infections. There is ongoing research into its effects on FIV, the feline form of HIV.

Pellitory causes hayfever in some people, and is called asthma weed in parts of Australia. It is declared a noxious weed there, which must be destroyed. Even in Britain, it is best avoided if you suffer allergies.

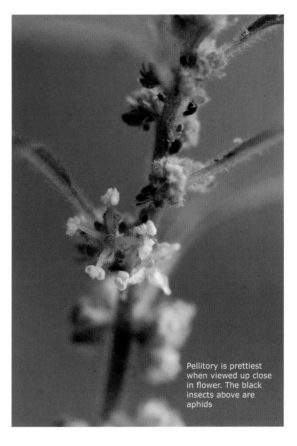

Pellitory is prettiest when viewed up close in flower. The black insects above are aphids

**Pellitory tea**
Harvest pellitory in the summer while it is flowering, breaking off a stem about halfway up (it snaps easily), leaving the rest to grow back. The fresh herb is considered to be the most effective, but it works well dried too.

Pour a cup of **boiling water** onto 2 teaspoons of the **chopped fresh** or 1 teaspoon of the **dried herb** and leave to infuse for 10–15 minutes. Add honey to taste (the tea is somewhat astringent).

**Dose:** Drink a cupful three times a day.

*Its action upon the urinary calculus is perhaps more marked than any other simple agent at present employed.*
– Mrs Grieve (1931)

**Pellitory tea**
• cystitis
• bladder irritation
• urinary gravel
• painful urination
• fluid retention

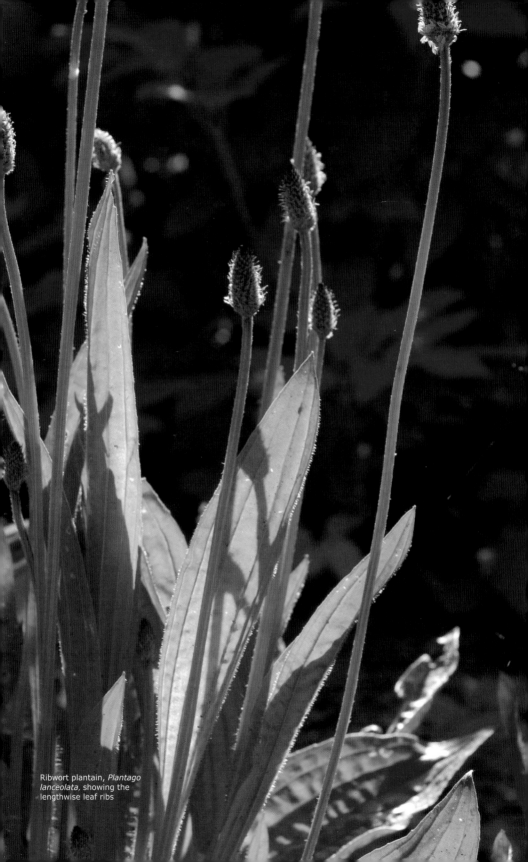

Ribwort plantain, *Plantago lanceolata*, showing the lengthwise leaf ribs

# Plantain *Plantago major, P. lanceolata*

**Common weeds of footpaths and lawns, the plantains were once celebrated as magical herbs in pre-Christian times, and have followed European settlers around the world.**

**Plantain is the best first-aid remedy for insect stings, and quickly deals with bites, cuts, and ulcers. It is widely available, safe to use and effective for a number of common ailments including old coughs, bronchitis, sore throats and irritable digestive tracts.**

Plantain is a plant now regarded primarily as a weed except by herbalists, but it had an illustrious past, being one of nine sacred herbs of the Anglo-Saxons, a "mother of worts." It had a reputation for clearing poisons, from bites as well as infections.

Plantains are found almost anywhere there is human habitation, though they have never had an economic value. Greater plantain in particular grows by preference on the compacted soils of paths and tracks, and seems to thrive on being downtrodden.

To Native Americans this plant became "white man's footprint", one that sprang up in the footsteps of the settlers. The plant's name *Plantago* itself comes from *planta* or sole of the foot.

The Anglo-Saxon name of plantain was *waybroed* or *waybrode*, later "waybread", because it grew by the way or path rather than because it made wonderful eating.

Plantains are familiar "weeds" in any lawn, and will return, even when cut often and short. The young leaves have a slightly bitter flavor from tannins, and though quite tough can be eaten in salads or as a spinach. They become bitter and more fibrous as they age. Buckshorn plantain is grown as a perennial salad crop in Italy and other parts of Europe.

Children all over the world use the flower heads of ribwort, as seen in the photo on the opposite page, as a sort of natural pop gun in the game "soldiers" or "kemps."

In Europe a piece of plantain root used to be carried in the pocket to protect against snakebite, but was no doubt more effective when actually applied to the wound as well as being ingested. The North American name snakeweed is an echo of that time.

## Use plantain for...
Ribwort is the number one field remedy for insect stings and bites.

**Plantaginaceae
Plantain family**

**Description:** Perennial plants with a rosette of ribbed leaves and wind-pollinated flowers on erect stalks.

**Habitat:** Footpaths, roadsides, waste ground, meadows, and lawns.

**Species used:** Greater plantain (*P. major*) and ribwort or narrowleaf plantain (*P. lanceolata*) are the main species used medicinally.

**Distribution:** Ribwort and greater plantain are found virtually everywhere with a temperate climate.

**Related species:** Buckshorn plantain (*P. coronopus*) is grown in Italy as a salad crop. There are around 250 species in the *Plantago* genus worldwide. Many of them have similar medicinal properties.

**Parts used:** Leaves, seeds, sometimes root.

Hoary plantain (*Planta-go media*) (right) is the most beautiful plantain, with pale lilac flowers

*Pliny records in the first century AD that 'Themison, a famous physician, sets forthe a whole booke of the hearbe waibred or plantaine, wherein he highly praiseth it; and challengeth it to himself the honour of first finding it out, notwithstanding it be a triviall and common hearbe trodden under everie man's foot.'*
– quoted in Gordon (1980)

**Running sore in ye Legge**
*Plantine water & oatmeal flour made into a plaster on the sore, wetting again with Plantine water and use plantine water to wash it.*
– Archdale Palmer's recipes 1659–72

*Indian bandaid.*
– a Cherokee elder's view of plantain

A crushed leaf rubbed onto the painful area will bring relief at once – it's almost miraculous.

Greater plantain also works for pain relief, but the leaves are tougher and not as juicy, so choose ribwort first if it is available. We find that any plantain, applied immediately, is effective for nettle stings and prefer it to dock leaf.

Plantain's antihistamine effect is also beneficial for hayfever and other allergies, and combines well as a tea with elderflower and mint. Plantain has long been a trusted plant for healing wounds (a vulnerary), and Shakespeare mentions it twice as a healer of broken shins. We haven't tried it on broken bones, but have found it to be very efficient at clearing heat and inflammation.

A patient of Julie's had deep red and painful shins from a radiation burn, and came every few days for several weeks for a dressing of fresh plantain juice mixed with slippery elm powder. Other fresh herbs such as chickweed and yarrow were added to the juice at times, but ribwort was the mainstay. The patient's legs healed and have not needed further treatment.

Julie also uses plantain poultices for the heat and swelling of varicose veins and varicose eczema.

Plantains are great purifiers, with an ability to draw dirt, pus and venom out of wounds. They have even been used to treat blood poisoning and gangrene. A poultice of crushed plantain leaves is the perfect remedy for the skinned knees of childhood, drawing out dirt while soothing and healing.

Abbé Kneipp (1821–97) characterized plantain's healing action thus:

*plantain closes the gaping wound with a seam of gold thread; for, just as gold will not admit of rust, so the plantain will not admit of rotting and gangrenous flesh.*

These same qualities make plantain useful for treating infections of the teeth and gums. Simply place a wad of plantain leaf against the affected area and back it up by plantain tea or tincture as a mouthwash. Plantain can be used to help relieve toothache until you can get to the dentist.

Plantain has a soothing effect on the mucous membranes of the digestive tract, and has been used successfully for stomach ulcers and irritable bowel complaints. The leaves stop the bleeding too, so are good for ulcerative colitis. The seeds are even more soothing than the leaf, but probably do not stop the bleeding as well.

The seeds can be eaten raw or cooked, and are very rich in vitamin B1. Ground into a meal and mixed with flour they can make a form of bread. The whole seeds can be boiled like sago, and have a pleasant mild flavor, but this is a bit fiddly and time-consuming.

The seed husks swell up and are very absorbent, providing a source of dietary fiber for constipation and other digestive disorders. It is not surprising that the mucilaginous and binding herb psyllium (or isaphagula) is from *Plantago ovata*, a close relative of our plantains and native to the Middle East and India. As well as being anti-diarrheal the mucilage in plantain is good for starching clothes.

Ribwort is the best of the plantains for treating coughs, and is recommended for chronic bronchitis as well as other persistent irritable coughs. It helps to bring up old stuck phlegm, and is particularly good for hot, dry coughs.

Greater or hoary plantain, having broader leaves, is better for hot, tired feet or plantar fasciitis. Do

as the Native Amerticans did and put the leaves in your shoes; keep there until the leaves dry out and then replace with fresh ones.

Plantain's long history has been benign. One exception came in a case of witchcraft in Scotland. In 1623 Bessie Smith confessed to treating "heart fevers" by giving "wayburn leaves" to take for nine mornings, with a charm. But was this worse than using plantain on St John's eve, as everyone did?

*It is the best herb for blood poisoning: reducing the swelling and completely healing a limb where poisoning has made amputation imminent.*
– Dr Christopher (1976)

*Plantago major* by Maria Merian (1717)

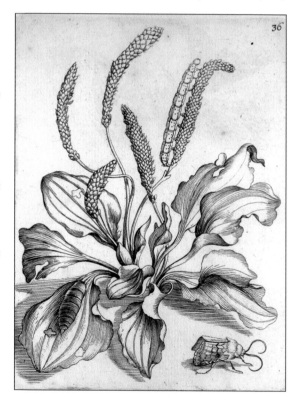

**LEAF**
**Leaf in shoe**
• plantar fasciitis
• tired feet

**Crushed leaf**
• insect bites & stings
• allergic rashes
• cuts and wounds
• infected cuts
• bleeding
• mouth ulcers
• boils and ulcers
• burns
• acne rosacea
• shingles

**Plantain tea,**
**Plantain tincture**
• coughs
• mild bronchitis
• irritable bowel
• hemorrhoids
• hay fever

**Plantain succus**
• coughs
• sore throats
• mild bronchitis
• irritable bowel
• stomach ulcers
• hay fever

**SEED**
• constipation
• irritable bowel

## Harvesting plantain

For first-aid use, plantain leaves can be picked and used whenever needed as they remain green through the year. Crush or chew, then apply. If you live in an area with harsh winters, you can freeze the leaves for winter use. For making a medicine to preserve, gather the leaves during the summer. To dry the leaves, spread them on brown paper or a drying screen in a warm dry place, turning the leaves daily until they are crisp. Discard if they go black.

Harvest the seeds when they are ripe, picking the heads and spreading them on brown paper to dry completely before stripping the seeds off for storage in brown paper bags or in jars.

## Plantain tea

Use a heaped teaspoonful of **crumbled dry leaf** or a **fresh leaf of plantain** per mugful of boiling water, and leave to infuse for ten minutes.

**Dose:** Drink a mugful three times a day.

## Plantain tincture

Pick **fresh plantain leaves** and put them in a blender with enough **vodka** to cover them. Blend to a green mush, and pour into a jar. Put in a cool dark place for a few days, then strain and bottle.

**Dose:** Half to one teaspoonful three times a day.

## Plantain succus

Juice **fresh plantain leaves** and mix the juice with an equal amount of **honey**. Pour into sterilized bottles and store in a cool place.

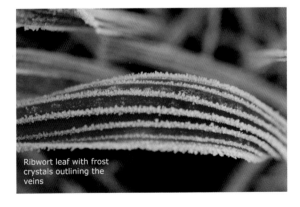
Ribwort leaf with frost crystals outlining the veins

**Dose:** 1 teaspoonful as needed for coughs (ribwort is best); 1 teaspoonful 3 times daily for stomach ulcers. Use externally a dressing, for ulcers and other sores.

## Plantain seed

The seeds and husks can be ground in a coffee grinder before use, or used whole.

**Dose:** 1 teaspoonful sprinkled on food, once to three times daily.

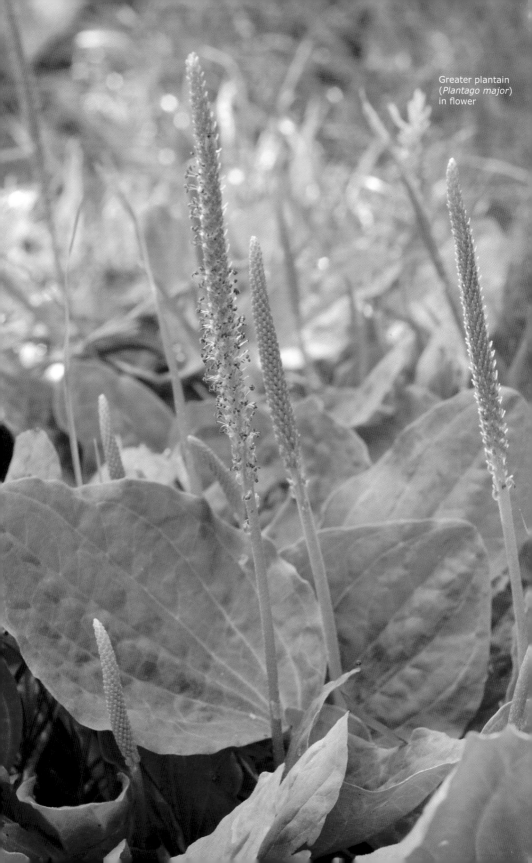

Greater plantain
(*Plantago major*)
in flower

# Ramsons, Bear garlic *Allium ursinum*

**Finding a swathe of ramsons (bear garlic) in a dark wood is one of the joys of early spring, with the bright green leaves and strong garlic smell tempting you to gather for the pot.**

**Liliaceae**
**Lily family**

**Description:** A bulb producing a carpet of greenery in damp wooded areas in spring, followed by beautiful white starry flowers in early summer. Up to 15" tall.

**Habitat:** Woodland, stream banks, and moist field sides.

**Distribution:** Widely distributed in the British Isles, Europe, and Asia. A garden plant in North America.

**Related species:** There are a number of *Allium* species found in North America that have similar uses to ramsons, including wild garlic (*A. canadense*) and the introduced field garlic (*A. vineale*). Use smell as your guide – if it smells strongly of garlic or onions, it is edible.

**Parts used:** Leaves, flowers, and sometimes bulbs.

*Let food be thy medicine and medicine be thy food.*
*– Hippocrates (460– 377 BC)*

**This is also a wonderful medicine for the digestive tract, and helps keep the heart and circulation healthy. Ramsons cleanses the body, balancing the gut flora, and is effective in removing infections.**

Ramsons has been a folk medicine favorite in Europe since the ancient Greeks, its uses in both kitchen and medicine cabinet matching those of its cultivated garlic cousin. Its unusual common name probably comes from an Old English word, *hramson*, which unsurprisingly meant wild garlic; its second Latin name of *ursinum*, or bear, perhaps relating to the smell, seems to have little relation to British experience (though see Mrs Grieve's gripes on the next page!).

You don't find this wonderful herb for sale in an herb or health shop, so you have to harvest your own. Luckily, it is usually abundant where it grows, carpeting woods and dells with its pungent greenery in the early spring.

Ramsons has similar medicinal properties to garlic, with the added benefit of being tolerated well by people who have problems with onions or garlic. We hope you find it as delicious as we do.

Gourmet cooks and posh restaurants extol the piquant flavor of fresh ramsons leaves, but it is also there for you to forage. The leaves can be eaten raw or cooked. Try them chopped and sprinkled on a variety of foods. A bright green garlic butter made from the leaves would be at home on a science fiction set, but is actually really tasty.

The bright white flowers can be used too, and are attractive and flavorsome sprinkled on salads. But note that once the flowers open, the palatability of the leaves decreases as they become harsher-tasting and less full-bodied.

## Use ramsons for...

Fresh ramsons eaten in spring is a gentle tonic for the whole body. By "cleansing the blood" it also helps with skin problems. Like ordinary garlic, ramsons improves the circulation and helps protect the heart. Better circulation assists

*Ramsons growing near High Force, Teesside, England, in May*

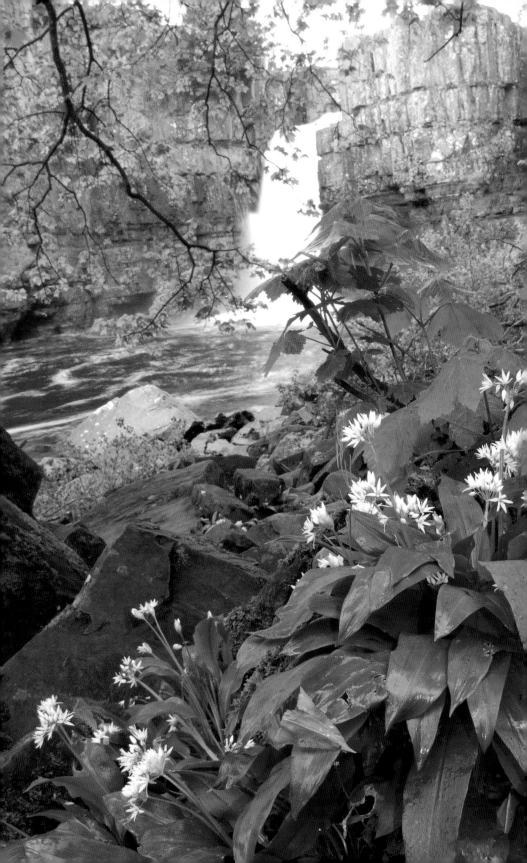

memory and eyesight, and will genrally lift the health.

You can make a poultice for boils and minor cuts by mashing a fresh ramsons leaf to place on them, holding it in place with a sticking plaster. Reapply a couple of times a day until healed. Ramsons is a good antibacterial and antifungal agent, though not as strong as ordinary garlic.

Ramsons is one of the best medicines for bowel problems. Julie has found in patients that it can settle a digestive tract that has never been quite right since a gut infection. Also, ramsons balances the gut flora, and is beneficial for ulcerative colitis, Crohn's disease, irritable bowel syndrome, chronic gastroenteritis, colic, and flatulence – in fact, it helps relieve most forms of intestinal unhappiness.

Ramsons is best used as a fresh seasonal food and medicine but can be preserved for later use. Garlic tincture doesn't sound very appealing, however! Many herbalists recommend taking ramsons juice, which is effective, but we'd much rather have a few tablespoons of ramsons pesto or sauce and enjoy taking our medicine as food (recipes below).

**Fresh ramsons leaf**
• spring tonic
• skin problems
• IBS
• gas and bloating
• chronic colitis
• ulcerative colitis
• Crohn's disease

**Fresh leaf poultice**
• boils
• cuts

**Ramsons pesto and sauce**
• spring tonic
• skin problems
• IBS
• gas and bloating
• chronic colitis
• ulcerative colitis
• Crohn's disease

### Harvesting ramsons

Ramsons leaves can be harvested as soon as they appear in spring, and are at their best before the flowers open. The flowers are tasty, sprinkled on salads and other food. The bulbs can also be eaten, but we prefer to leave them to grow again the next year. Ramsons are locally abundant, so you should be able to harvest and preserve plenty of leaves without needing to disturb the bulbs.

### Ramsons pesto

Put **ramsons leaves** and enough **olive oil** to cover them in a blender. Blend until smooth. This vivid green sauce can be eaten fresh with pasta just like the more familiar Italian pesto made with basil and garlic. You can alter the taste by adding chopped pine nuts or sunflower seeds and freshly grated pecorino cheese. It is delicious spooned onto savory foods and can be added to salad dressings. This pesto can be frozen in small batches for use throughout the year.

### Ramsons sauce

Another way to preserve **ramsons** is to blend as above, but use 1 part **cider** or **white wine vinegar** to 3 parts **olive oil** as the liquid. The vinegar helps preserve the ramsons, and a jar of this will keep well in the fridge for months if it doesn't get eaten before then!

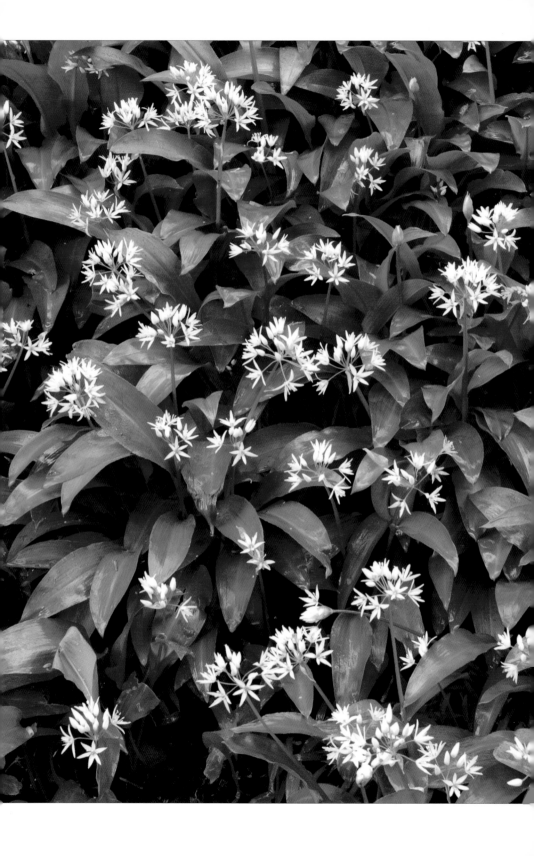

# Raspberry *Rubus idaeus*

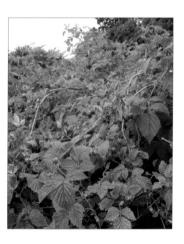

**Rosaceae
Rose family**

**Description:** A slender shrub, up to 6 feet high, with arching stems; less spiny and more delicate than blackberry canes. The leaves are a light green, and silvery underneath. The stems are bare in winter.

**Habitat:** Wild raspberries are often found growing along the edges of woods and forests.

**Distribution:** Found throughout North America, northern Europe, and northern Asia.

**Related species:** The North American grayleaf red raspberry (*R.idaeus* spp. *strigosus*) can be used interchangeably with the Old World species. In China, Korean bramble (*R. coreanus*) fruit is used as a kidney and liver tonic.

**Parts used:** Leaves and berries.

Generally known as red raspberry in North America, raspberry leaf tea is well recognized for strengthening the uterus prior to childbirth, and for relieving painful periods. It is also an effective and soothing remedy for flu and fevers, helping reduce the aches and pains that go with them.

This tea is a good source of readily assimilated calcium and other minerals, making it a health-enhancing alternative to regular tea. Raspberries, especially wild ones, are very high in salvestrols, a class of cancer-fighting chemicals.

Raspberry is a member of the rose family, a plant of the Old World, spreading out to the temperate regions from the Mediterranean. The second part of its name, "idaeus," refers to this ancient origin.

The Greek version of the raspberry legend concerns Ida, daughter of the King of Crete. One day she was looking after her infant, Jupiter, while picking berries on a mountainside. The lusty babe made so much noise that Ida was distracted. When she pricked herself her blood caused what were white berries to turn red. They have remained so ever since – and still grow on the slopes of Mt Ida in modern Crete.

Raspberry was given the common name "raspis," meaning rough or hairy fruit (by contrast with the blackberry), and also "hindberry" because female deer would feed on the leaves, and thereby assist in their own birthing.

The noted animal herbalist Juliette de Baïracli Levy has long advocated dog breeders using raspberry leaf tea, with impressive whelping results throughout the world. She quotes a Romany source: "Let all creatures with young, human and animal, take freely of raspberry herb. They will have very easy 'times' and will be saved a tremendous amount of suffering."

## Use raspberry for…

The best way to enjoy wild raspberries is to eat them straight off the bush. They may not be as large as the commercial and garden varieties, but the deep, satisfying flavor is special. As the English herbalist John Parkinson wrote in 1629: "The berries are eaten in the Summertime, as an afternoones dish, to please the taste of the sicke as well as the sound."

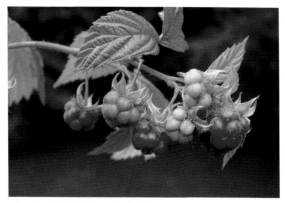

But it is the leaves rather than the berries that have the most benefit medicinally. The best time to pick them is on a sunny morning after the dew has dried off. Most herbals say drying the leaves is best, but we find the fresh and dried alternatives equally good.

If you are drying the leaves to use later, hang up bunches of the canes tied together with string, or spread the leaves on a drying rack – a linen cupboard is an ideal place. When they are crisp, they can be packed away in brown paper bags or bottles for storage.

Raspberry leaf is astringent, meaning that it tightens and tones tissue. It is high in nutrients, including iron, manganese, and calcium.

The leaf tea is mainly used in pregnancy to help ease delivery and reduce pain in labor. Julie drank it when she was pregnant, and while she wouldn't say labor was easy (the very name means work, after all!) it was not painful. Raspberry leaf continues its work after the baby is born, by helping the uterus return to normal and promoting milk production.

You may find disagreement in various books about how long to use raspberry leaf in pregnancy. Some authors advise taking it throughout while others restrict it to the last two or three months only. It partly depends on the dose, and we suggest you follow what your midwife or herbalist says is best for you personally.

Many herbals recommend using an ounce of dried leaf per pint of water, but this is a very strong brew and isn't too pleasant to drink. Unless you are trying to stop diarrhea, this strength isn't necessary. We think a weaker tea taken more often is a better idea.

As well as pregnancy and for periods, raspberry tea and vinegar can be used to counter anemia, and to relieve colds, flu, and diarrhea. See the recipes overleaf.

**Raspberries** are high in vitamin C and other antioxidants. They are also high in a newly discovered class of chemicals called **salvestrols**, which have proven anti-cancer activity.

Professor Gerry Potter, Head of Medicinal Chemistry at De Montfort University and Director of the Cancer Drug Discovery Group, recommends a diet of foods that are naturally high in salvestrols, which includes raspberries and other red and blue berries.

Recent research has found that agrochemicals inhibit plants from producing salvestrols, so wild or organically grown plants have higher levels. Here's another reason to enjoy your wild raspberries!

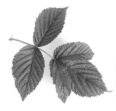

**Raspberry leaf tea**
• childbirth
• lactation
• heavy menstruation
• anemia
• flu
• muscle cramps
• osteoporosis
• diarrhea
• nausea

**Other uses for raspberry leaf tea**
• as a mouthwash for mouth ulcers and gum problems
• as a gargle for sore throats
• when cool as a soothing eyewash for sore and irritated eyes
• as a healing wash for cuts and abrasions

**Raspberry vinegar**
• colds & flu
• sore throats
• digestion
• arthritis
• salad dressing

**Raspberry oxymel**
• sore throats
• colds & flu
• sluggish digestion
• arthritis

### Raspberry leaf tea

Pour a cupful of **boiling water** onto 1 rounded tablespoonful of dried **raspberry leaf** or a handful of fresh leaves. Let it brew for 15 minutes, then strain and drink, either hot or cold.

**Dosages:** For general use, drink 1 cupful one to three times a day.

In the last two/three months of pregnancy and for several weeks after giving birth, drink two cups daily, or as instructed by your herbal practitioner or midwife. To normalize heavy periods, drink 3 cups a day during your period, and 1 cup a day the rest of the month. At the first sign of a cold or flu, stop eating for a day or two and drink lots of raspberry leaf tea.

For diarrhea, make a stronger infusion with 2 to 3 teaspoonfuls of dried leaf per cup of boiling water. Drink 1 cupful three times a day. Children can have a wineglassful, and babies a teaspoonful.

### Raspberry vinegar

Fill a jam jar with freshly picked **raspberries** and pour in enough **cider vinegar** to cover them. Cover the jar and put it in a warm place such as a sunny windowsill, shaking it every few days.

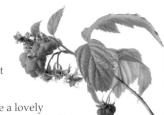

After two weeks the vinegar should be a lovely deep pink. Strain through a jelly bag or fine sieve. If you want a clear vinegar, don't press the pulp – just let the liquid drip out – otherwise squeeze to get the most flavor out of your raspberries, and pour into a sterile bottle.

**Dosage:** Take 1 teaspoonful every few hours for colds and flu.

This rich, sweet-sour vinegar can also be used to bring a touch of summer sunshine to winter salad dressings. It has a wonderful flavor, enjoyed in the best gourmet restaurants – and your own home.

### Raspberry oxymel

Mix equal parts of **honey** and **raspberry vinegar**.

**Dosage:** For sore throats, use 1 tablespoon as a gargle before swallowing. For a sluggish digestive system, add 1 tablespoon of the oxymel to a mug of hot water, and drink before meals.

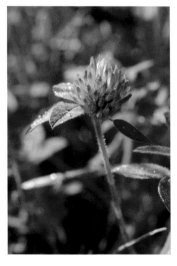

# Red clover *Trifolium pratense*

**An important nitrogen-fixing forage crop, red clover is also a significant medicinal plant with a long history as a blood cleanser. It is used for chronic constipation, skin complaints, chronic degenerative diseases, and bronchitis. It has been included in many anti-cancer formulae, and helps balance hormone levels during the menopause, relieving symptoms such as hot flashes.**

**Fabaceae (Leguminosae) Pea family**

**Description:** A common perennial with purplish-red flowers and a single pale chevron on the leaves.

**Habitat:** Grassland, roadsides.

**Distribution:** Native and also cultivated throughout Europe; naturalized in the Americas, Australia, and many other places.

**Related species:** The other common species is white clover (*T. repens*), with medicinal uses similar to those of red clover. There are over 200 species of clover worldwide.

**Parts used:** Flower heads with upper leaves, collected in early summer.

Clover or trefoil (three leaves) has a sacred past. It had significance for the Druids, and St Patrick was said to have used a clover in the meadow to explain the Trinity to Irish pagans. As befitted a plant of such fortunate lineage clover was worthy, with other holy herbs, to protect the virtuous against dark forces. One old rhyme went (in Sir Walter Scott's 1815 version):

*Trefoil, vervain, St John's wort, dill,
Hinder witches of their will.*

The oldest form of the name "clover" we have is Anglo-Saxon *cloeferwort*, the last syllable being a marker of its herbal value (a "wort" is a medicinal herb). The name may have derived from the Latin *clava* or club, probably the three-knotted club of Hercules; from the fourteenth century clover was the symbol of the card suit "clubs."

In Tudor times the plant was called *claver*, which later became *clover*. The Irish national flower, the shamrock, means "small clover," though it's really an *Oxalis*.

In the Middle Ages legumes, like peas, beans, and vetches, were grown as fodder and food crops. From the mid-seventeenth century farmers added red and white clover; only much later did scientists learn why it was so useful: clover fixed organic nitrogen in the soil in its root nodules. Clover remains an excellent hay (to be "in clover" still means to have abundance).

*Red clover is wonderful for scrofulous and skin diseases, as an antidote to cancer, and for bronchitis and spasmodic affections.*
– Dr Christopher (1976)

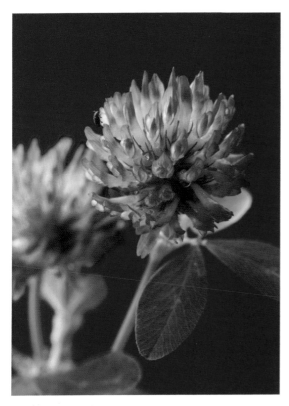

*Red clover seldom cures cancer, but it fairly reliably will cause a membrane to grow around the tumor and contain it, which is helpful, especially if followed by surgery. This has especially been observed in breast cancer.*
– Wood (2008)

## Use red clover for…

The best-known use of all for clover is of course the luck of finding a rare four-leafed one. In some folk traditions, the three leaves represented faith, hope, and charity (love), and the fourth was God's grace; in everyday terms, it meant luck. Nowadays you can order a plastic-sealed lucky four-leaved clover online (some sites offer organically grown ones). Who gets the luck, one wonders – probably the seller.

Your luck may be more certain if you use clover herbally. Red clover works gently to improve elimination over a wide front, helping the body rid itself of toxins by increasing the flow of urine, moving mucus out of the lungs, increasing the flow of bile, and acting as a gentle laxative.

This slow and steady action plus its high content of trace minerals means that red clover is effective for a wide range of health problems, and is gentle enough for children. Clover is most effective when taken consistently for several months for chronic conditions such as skin problems.

Its ability to remove waste products, combined with a capacity to prevent the formation of abnormal cells, underlies clover's old reputation for treating cancers, including breast, prostate, and lymphatic forms. As with all claims for treating cancer, this has been controversial. One US pioneer of plant-

Also, clover is beloved of bees and yields wonderful honey (the white clover is superior), and the white form, with a mass of roots, gives a fine lawn – though clover lawns are currently unfashionable.

In terms of culinary uses, clover leaves and flowers can be eaten in salads, and the seeds soaked and sprouted. Clover wine is well-liked. The dried flowers are mixed with coltsfoot leaves as an herbal tobacco or used as a snuff.

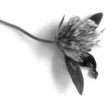

based cancer remedies, Harry Hoxsey, had red clover as the main herb in his formula, and it has been used in many others.

Red clover's soothing expectorant effect is beneficial in treating coughs and bronchitis, and the plant remains official in the *British Herbal Pharmacopoeia* as an anti-inflammatory.

Red clover's ability to alleviate menopausal symptoms is related to its flavonoid content. Flavonoids are estrogen-like plant chemicals (or phyto-estrogens)

that help maintain normal estrogen levels during menopause, providing relief for hot flashes. However, red clover is safe to use and beneficial in cases of breast cancer because it reduces high estrogen levels (see box on right).

Red clover itself does not have a blood-thinning effect but the coumarin it contains can convert to dicoumarol, which is a blood thinner, if the plants ferment on drying. If dried quickly, this will not occur, but clover should not be used in quantity by anyone taking blood-thinning medication.

---

**Phyto-estrogens**

Phyto-estrogens can exert an estrogenic effect in the body, which is useful in the menopause when estrogen levels are low. What is less well known is the fact that they can also exert an anti-estrogenic effect in the body.

This is because phyto-estrogens have a weaker estrogenic effect than estrogens produced by the body, and both bind to estrogen receptor sites. If estrogen levels are high, the weaker plant estrogens reduce the overall estrogenic effect, which is one reason why red clover is beneficial in breast cancer treatment.

---

### Harvesting red clover

Pick the flowers and top leaves in early summer (the flowers growing in autumn are not as sweet) when the morning dew has dried off. Choose newly opened pink flowers. Dry thoroughly, spreading them out on paper or trays, no more than one flowerhead deep, in a warm dry place away from direct sunlight. When fully dried they are crumbly to the touch. Store in glass bottles away from the light to maintain the red color.

### Red clover tea

Use 1 or 2 heaped teaspoons of dried red clover flowers per cup or mug of boiling water and allow to infuse for ten minutes. Strain and drink.

**Dose:** 3 or 4 cups a day. Can be taken by children. For chronic toxicity, constipation and skin problems this tea needs to be taken consistently over a period of five or six weeks, as the effect is cumulative. To help with hot flashes, it is best drunk cold at the first onset of a flash.

### Red clover and curled dock tincture

Put roughly equal amounts of **red clover blossom** and chopped **curled dock root** in a jar, and pour in enough **vodka** to cover the herbs. Leave in a dark place for two weeks, then strain. Pour the liquid into clean bottles and label.

**Dose:** Half a teaspoon 2 to 3 times daily.

---

**Red clover tea**
• chronic constipation
• acne
• eczema
• psoriasis
• swollen glands
• hot flashes
• coughs
• bronchitis

**Red clover & curled dock tincture**
• chronic constipation
• toxicity
• acne
• eczema
• psoriasis
• swollen glands

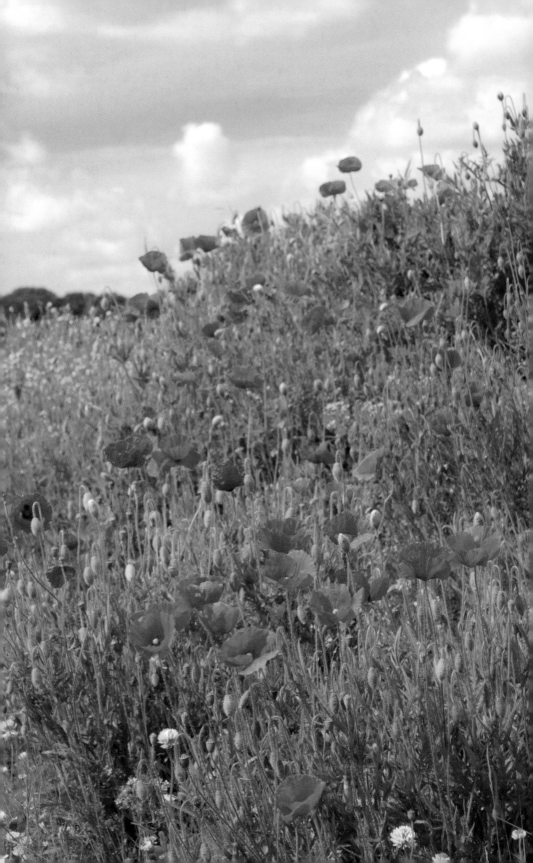

# Red poppy *Papaver rhoeas*

**Red poppy is an archetypal weed of summer, flowering in profusion on disturbed soil and among unsprayed crops. Unwanted by farmers, it has long been a useful country herbal remedy. Red poppy is soothing and sedative, relieves pain and helps sleep, but without the narcotic effects of its relative, the opium poppy.**

The poppy has always had a powerful hold on human imagination, and not just in opium dreams. Everybody in Britain knows "poppy day," held in memory of the sacrifice made by millions in the First World War and since. Yet poppy is also symbolically the plant of forgetfulness and sleep. In some cultures it has been a plant of fertility, with its vast production of seeds and vivid red petals a reminder of the blood of life and of war, as also of renewal and rebirth.

As befits a plant of life, death, blood, dream, and sleep, poppy coincides with man's many civilizations, and its own history is intertwined in them. It is as old as agriculture itself, growing in and alongside the earliest grain crops.

Yet British fields have not always been scarlet with poppies as the grain ripens through a hot summer. It's well within memory that the fields and hedgerows lacked virtually any poppies and other once common wild plants. Why? Because we have endured a fertilizer, herbicide, and insecticide bombardment of heroic propor-

tions. The pace has only dropped in the past twenty to thirty years. Policy-makers have now rediscovered the value of leaving land fallow and of field margins, and have paid farmers to do it. Presto! the poppies have duly come back, especially where fields have been left unsprayed.

One of poppy's characteristics is that it looks and feels fragile, its stem being thin and wobbly, its gossamer-fine petals falling off to the touch, whereas in reality it is tailor-made for survival. Its flowering season is long, through the summer. Calculations have shown that each mature plant produces some 17,000 tiny seeds a year, which can sit in a state of dormancy for fifty or more years, awaiting the right conditions.

A change such as new ploughing or deep trenches being dug will release forgotten poppy seeds and give them the disturbed ground they need to flourish *en masse*. Hence the shock when poppies suddenly flowered amid the killing fields of the Great War. This stark contrast led to a Canadian

**Papaveraceae**
**Poppy family**

**Description:** An annual with bright red flowers, growing to about 2 feet. Flowers most of the summer.

**Habitat:** Farmland and other disturbed ground.

**Distribution:** Native to Europe, naturalized in much of North America.

**Related species:** Long-headed poppy (*P. dubium*) is very similar but has paler petals and long seed capsules. Opium poppy (*P. somniferum*) is a larger plant with gray–green leaves and the flowers are usually pale lilac with darker centers.

**Parts used:** Flowers and seeds, harvested in summer.

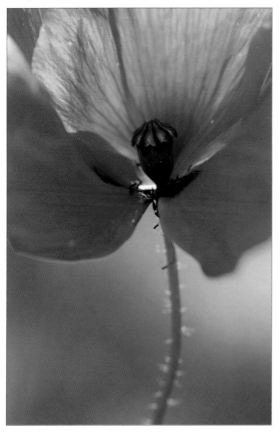

November, solemn services are held for the fallen of all wars. Participants and many besides all wear red poppies made of paper.

It is worth underlining here that our focus is on the red poppy and not the opium poppy. Opium poppies have been grown domestically in England for millennia, and 150 years ago went into laudanum (a tincture in alcohol) and paregoric elixir (a camphorated extract). Modern pain-relieving medications including morphine and codeine are derived from opium poppy, but are prescription-only.

### Use red poppy for...

Red poppy doesn't have the dangerous reputation of its infamous cousin. Taking red poppy herbally is non-addictive and generally safe: its weak opiates work well medicinally but are not in strong enough concentration to do harm.

Red poppy has long been familiar in British country traditions. For example, the petals were collected as a coloring agent for wines and other herbal remedies. Indeed, the petals are still used to add color to sweets and some herbal teas.

Red poppy petals can be added to summer salads for brightness, and the seeds collected as a topping for bread and to use in cooking. The seeds have mild sedative qualities.

Our glycerite recipe is good for coughs, nervous digestion, anxiety, and insomnia. It is gentle and safe

*Boil poppy heads in ale; let the patient drink it, and he will sleep.*
*– The Physicians of Myddfai (13th century)*

*The Flowers cool, and asswage Pain, and dispose to Sleep. ...*
*– Pechey (1707)*

medical orderly, John McCrae, finding time between his terrible duties at Ypres in 1915 to write the poem "In Flanders Fields." He posted it to a magazine in London. It was printed and soon became immensely popular worldwide.

The poem and its powerful link to an archetypal plant of war inspired the British Legion (now the Royal British Legion) after the armistice to take up the call of remembrance. Since then, on Remembrance Day each 11th of

for children who are over-excited and cannot sleep. The petals can also be made into a tincture that will tackle similar conditions.

In general, red poppy acts as a mild sedative that also promotes perspiration, soothes respiratory passages, and calms the system. Being slightly astringent, it helps remove excess mucus and improves the digestion. It soothes itchy or sore throats and hacking coughs. For insomnia, it combines well with lime blossom, wood betony, and vervain, and can also be used with hops and wild lettuce.

Red poppy is a great plant of myth and archetype, with medicinal virtues on a more humble scale for the home medicine cabinet.

### Red poppy glycerite

Fill a jar about three-quarters full of a mixture of 60% **vegetable glycerine** and 40% **water**. Add **poppy petals** to fill the jar, stirring so that the petals are covered in the glycerine mixture. Put the lid on the jar and place it in a sunny spot in the garden or on a window sill.

One of the little plastic inserts used by jam makers to keep the material pushed down under the surface of the liquid is handy, but if you don't have one just shake the jar or stir the contents every day. This will keep the petals from floating on the top. Once the petals have faded to white, usually after only a few days, they can be removed and fresh ones added over the summer until your liquid is a rich deep red color. It can then be strained, bottled and labeled. Your glycerite should keep well in a cool dark place until next year when you can make a fresh batch.

The glycerite is particularly good for children, as it doesn't contain alcohol and they will like the sweet taste. It is also good for coughs and irritable or nervous digestive tracts.

### Red poppy tincture

Fill a jar with **fresh poppy petals**, then top it up with **vodka**. Put the lid on and shake well, adding a little more vodka if needed to fill the jar. Place the jar in a cool dark place – a cupboard is perfect – for two weeks, then strain and bottle.

The alcohol in a tincture makes it more warming and dispersing. While the uses are much the same as for the glycerite, the tincture is probably better for pain as it is more rapidly absorbed and has a quicker effect.

You can also combine your tincture and glycerite half and half, reducing the sweetness of the glycerite and making the tincture taste better.

**Red poppy glycerite**
- insomnia
- irritable cough
- nervous digestion
- IBS
- headache
- over-excitability
- anxiety
- nervousness

**Red poppy tincture**
- insomnia
- nervous digestion
- IBS
- headache
- over-excitability
- anxiety
- nervousness

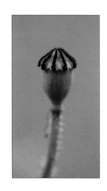

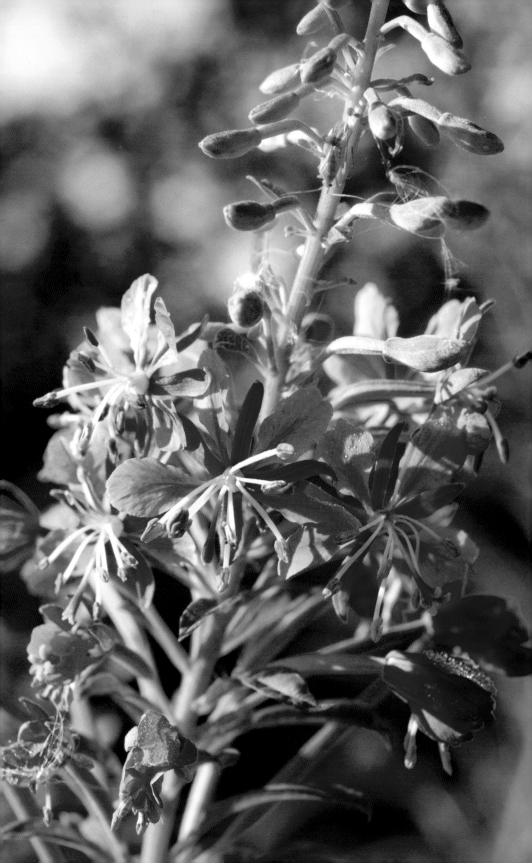

# Rosebay willowherb, Fireweed

*Chamerion angustifolium* syn. *Epilobium angustifolium, Chamaenerion angustifolium*

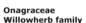

**This beautiful native plant is stunning enough to be grown in any garden and yet is considered a weed. It has not been used much in medicine in recent years but was a favorite of the American Eclectic physicians in treating diarrhea and typhoid. Its soothing, astringent, and tonic action is wonderful for all sorts of intestinal irritation, and it makes a good mouthwash.**

**Onagraceae
Willowherb family**

**Description:** A tall, 4 to 5 foot high perennial, with stunning magenta flower spikes in summer and into fall.

**Habitat:** Heaths, mountains, forest clearings, waste ground, and railway embankments.

**Distribution:** Across northern Europe, Asia, and North America; also parts of north Africa.

**Related species:** Rosebay willowherb is closely related to other willowherbs in the *Epilobium* genus: see page 186.

**Parts used:** Flower spikes and leaves, harvested in summer.

Rosebay willowherb is one of Europe's largest and most beautiful wildflowers. In North America, it is called fireweed because of its tendency to spring up as an early pioneer on burnt land. It is rarely grown in gardens these days, except for the rare white form.

Julie remembers the excitement of seeing her first fireweed as she and her parents drove north on the Alaska Highway, when she was eleven. We've heard of one American herbalist who cheers every time she sees fireweed by the roadside, sometimes drawing strange looks. It's a plant that brings joy just by being there.

Rosebay willowherb is one of the first plants to appear whenever the earth is scarred. In Second World War Britain, it sprang up on bomb sites in London and elsewhere, rising like a phoenix from the ashes and rubble (its seeds last for years in a dormant state). In Clydebank, Scotland, it colonized the bombed Singer sewing machine factory site and was nicknamed Singerweed.

The "narrow leaves" (the English version of *angustifolium*) of the plant do resemble willow enough to earn its common name, but there is no real connection, medicinal or otherwise.

In Russia, the leaves are drunk as a tea called *kapoori*, while in Alaska the flowers are a valuable source of nectar for honey, and are made into jellies and syrups. This honey is said to be the most northerly available anywhere.

Various groups of native North Americans have used rosebay as a food plant. Supposedly the young shoots boiled in the spring taste like asparagus, but we haven't tried it, and "wild food" expert Roger Phillips is not a fan, as the attached quotation suggests.

### Use rosebay for...

The plant's astringency, however, works well in our syrup recipe, which is good for diarrhea and a pleasant remedy for children (and adults) who are suffering digestive upsets.

*Despite all the exotic tales of eating rosebay willow-herb I have been unable to make it palatable. It is far too bitter to enjoy as any kind of vegetable.*
*– Phillips (1983)*

*That it has not attained prominence as a remedy is not the fault of the plant, for in certain cases of summer bowel troubles it is without an equal.*
*– King's American Dispensatory (1898)*

*[Rosebay] Cleanses old patterns from the body and stimulates renewal of energies on all levels of being; attracts restorative healing energy from our surroundings.*
*– Rudd (1998)*

America's Eclectic doctors of a century and more ago favored rosebay willowherb for all kinds of diarrhea and enteritis, cholera infantum, or typhoid dysentery. *King's American Dispensatory* (1898) said of one of the leading Eclectics: "With Prof. Scudder, infusion of epilobium was a favorite remedy to correct and restrain the diarrhea of typhoid or enteric fever." The Eclectics also used the leaf infusion for uterine bleeding and heavy periods, and the fresh leaves as a poultice for "foul and indolent ulcers." We have found it works well for mouth ulcers.

Contemporary American herbalist David Winston uses rosebay to treat candida overgrowth.

Several flower essence makers produce a fireweed essence, saying it is a powerful aid in connecting us to the healing energies of nature and the earth. This helps in problems concerning change and in shifting stagnant energy patterns. It is used both for a "burnt-out" feeling and for shock and trauma. If you'd like to try making your own essence, follow the instructions given on page 154 for self-heal essence.

**Rosebay poultice**
• ulcers
• minor wounds

**Rosebay leaf tea**
• digestion
• diarrhea
• IBS
• heavy periods
• mouth ulcers
• sore throats
• prostate problems

**Rosebay syrup**
• diarrhea
• loose bowels
• childhood diarrhea

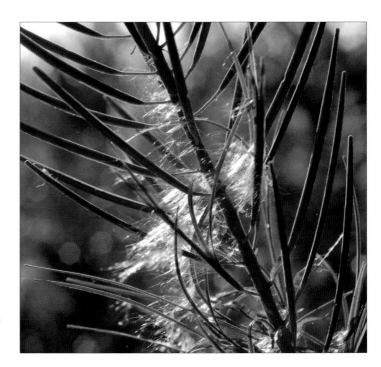

The fine, downy seeds of rosebay willowherb blow far and wide on the wind.

### Rosebay willowherb leaf poultice

The fresh leaves can be crushed and applied as a poultice to help minor wounds heal. Hold the leaves on with a plaster, and change for fresh crushed leaves a couple of times a day until healed. The early American Eclectic doctors found it effective for old ulcers.

### Rosebay willowherb tea

The leaves can be harvested in the spring or while the plant is in flower in the summer, and dried for use throughout the year. To dry, spread the leaves on paper in a shady place, turning them occasionally until crisp.

Use 3 or 4 **leaves** per cup of **boiling water** and infuse for about 5 minutes. Drink frequently for diarrhea, or use as a substitute for ordinary tea.

Can be used as a mouthwash for mouth ulcers and a gargle for sore throats.

### Rosebay willowherb syrup
**20 flower heads**
**2 cups water**

Bring to a boil and simmer until the color leaves the blossoms, in about 5–10 minutes. Strain the juice, return to the pot.

Add **4 oz sugar** to the reduced fluid, and **juice of a lemon.**

This turns the pale color a bright pink, almost like the blossoms you start with. Boil for 5 minutes, allow to cool a little, then bottle and label.

It will keep in the fridge for a few months.

This is a pleasant remedy for childhood diarrhea, and can be used for any case of intestinal irritation associated with loose bowels.

**Dose:** A dessertspoonful for children and a tablespoonful for adults, every few hours as needed.

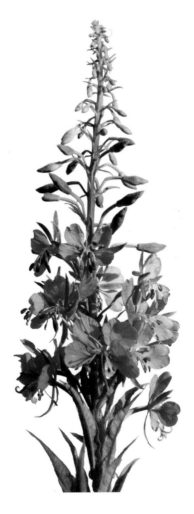

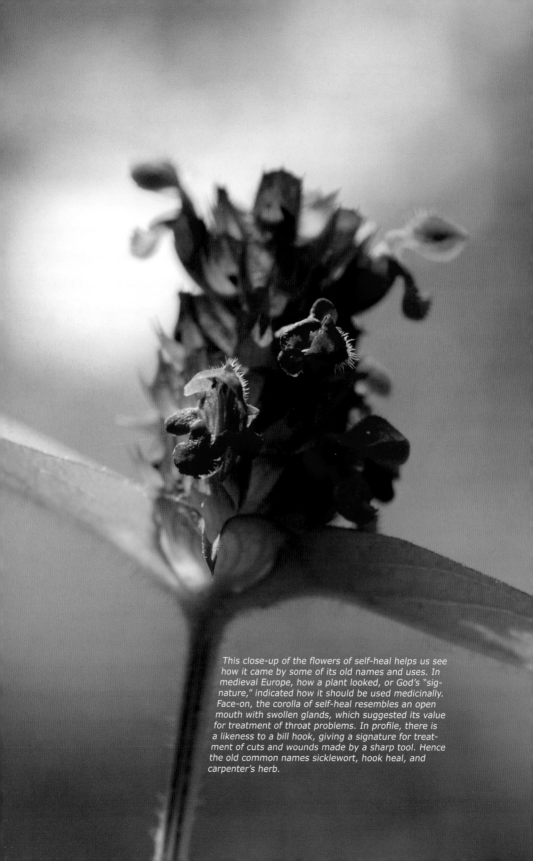

This close-up of the flowers of self-heal helps us see how it came by some of its old names and uses. In medieval Europe, how a plant looked, or God's "signature," indicated how it should be used medicinally. Face-on, the corolla of self-heal resembles an open mouth with swollen glands, which suggested its value for treatment of throat problems. In profile, there is a likeness to a bill hook, giving a signature for treatment of cuts and wounds made by a sharp tool. Hence the old common names sicklewort, hook heal, and carpenter's herb.

# Self-heal *Prunella vulgaris*

**Also called all-heal, self-heal was mentioned in Chinese medical literature of the Han dynasty (206 BC to AD 23), and is still used in Traditional Chinese Medicine. It was popular for centuries in Europe as a wound herb and for throat problems.**

**Self-heal has gained recent respect for its antiviral qualities. Effective for feverish colds and flu, it has also been proposed for treating herpes and AIDS, and is an underrated liver, gallbladder, and thyroid remedy.**

As you would expect from a plant known as all-heal, self-heal has a wide range of medicinal actions. It is, however, underused in contemporary western herbal medicine.

Self-heal has a long history of western folk use. One name it acquired was "touch and heal," indicating its value as first aid for cuts and wounds. It was also found to staunch bleeding and help knit a wound together. Taken internally as a tea, it treated fevers, diarrhea, and internal bleeding.

The Latin name *Prunella* was given by Linnaeus to *Brunella*, the German name of the plant. This reflected its use for "die Braüne" or quinsy, meaning a throat abscess. A self-heal tea was taken internally, and a self-heal mouthwash and gargle used to treat a wide range of mouth and throat problems.

In the European tradition the plant is picked just before or while flowering, but in China the flower tops are collected in late summer when they are starting to wither. This variation in time of harvesting, along with regional variations in the plant's chemistry, could explain the different uses of self-heal in the two traditions.

In Chinese medicine, self-heal is given for ascending liver fire and liver deficiency. It clears liver congestion and stagnation and brightens the eyes, which are regarded as linked to the liver. In common with European use, it is said to lessen heat and dissipate nodules, particularly in the neck, such as scrofula, lipoma, swollen glands, and goitre.

## Use self-heal for...
Julie has always used self-heal in her practice, mainly for treating flu and hot flashes. We knew we needed to take a deeper look at this plant when it seeded itself with exuberance all over our garden while we were writing this book – it seemed to be trying to

**Lamiaceae (Labiatae) Deadnettle family**

**Description:** A creeping perennial with downy leaves and violet flowers, reaching up to a foot tall.

**Habitat:** Lawns, meadows, and woods.

**Distribution:** Found virtually worldwide in temperate areas. Widespread in North America.

**Related species:** Cut-leaved self-heal (*P. laciniata*) has creamy white flowers and is found on dry lime soils.

**Parts used:** Flowers and leaves, dry flower spikes.

tell us something. The more we thought about and used self-heal, the more impressed we became.

Recent studies have shown self-heal to be an effective remedy for herpes. If we look back at the old herbals, we see this is not new. In 1640, John Parkinson wrote that self-heal "juice mixed with a little Hony of Roses, clenseth and healeth all ulcers and sores in the mouth and throate, and those also in the secret parts." We know today that both roses and self-heal have antiviral properties.

Self-heal is a good remedy for flu and fevers because it combines cooling, immune-stimulating, and antiviral qualities. It has been found to be effective against a broad range of bacteria, including *Mycobacterium tuberculi*, which causes tuberculosis.

The old use for goitre ties in with American herbalist James Duke's research on self-heal. He found it to be among the most effective herbs for hypothyroidism (underactive thyroid), which often leads to a goitre formation. He has also confirmed that self-heal treats Graves' disease and other hyperactive thyroid conditions. This means its effect is amphoteric, that is, it normalizes function by stimulating an underactive gland or reducing overactivity.

Self-heal is high on Duke's list of plants with marked antioxidant activity. Studies show that self-heal has strong immune-stimulatory effects, and calms inflammatory and allergic responses. In preventing viruses from replicating, it shows promise in the treatment of AIDS. It is also used for diabetes and high blood pressure.

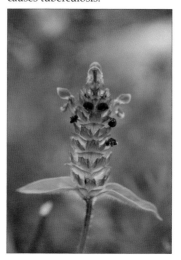 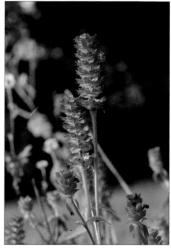

Self-heal ready for picking: in European medicine (left); in Chinese medicine (right).

### Self-heal tea

For tea, we prefer to harvest the flower spikes when they have finished flowering and are turning brown, drying naturally on the plant. You can shake out any ripe seeds to sow, ensuring a supply of plants for the years ahead.

Use about two **flower spikes** per mug of **boiling water** and infuse for 5 to 10 minutes. Drink freely. For hot flashes, it is best drunk cool. It can be used as a mouthwash and gargle for mouth ulcers and sore throats.

### Self-heal infused oil

Fill a jar with **fresh self-heal blossoms and leaves**. Pour **olive oil** in to fill the jar, stirring as you do so to allow air bubbles to escape. Cover the jar with a piece of cloth held on with a rubber band – this will allow any moisture to evaporate. Place the jar on a sunny window sill.

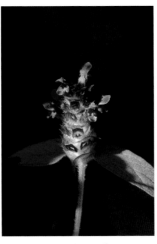

Check the jar every few days, and if necessary push the plant material back down under the surface of the oil. After two to four weeks the color will have drained out of the plants. Strain off the oil. Allow it to settle, so that any water will sink to the bottom, then pour the oil carefully into bottles and label. This oil will keep for several years, but it is best to make a fresh batch every summer if you can.

### Self-heal cream

To make a cream, you will be using some of the **self-heal oil** you have made, and combining it with a strong **self-heal tea**. This cream recipe can be used for other herbs or combinations of herbs too.

**2 fl oz oil**
**3/4 ounce beeswax**
**2 fl oz tea**

Put the oil and beeswax in one bowl and the infusion in another, and stand them both in a large pan of hot water. Heat until the beeswax melts. It is important that they are both the same temperature. Slowly pour the tea into the oil mixture while beating with an electric mixer set at the slowest speed. If you want, you can add a few drops of **self-heal stock essence** (instructions on next page). Once all the oil is mixed in and the mixture has emulsified and thickened, pour the cream into clean jars. Once set, label, and store in a cool place or in the fridge.

**Self-heal tea**
- general well-being
- fevers
- flu & viral infections
- mouth ulcers
- thyroid disorders
- throat problems

**Self-heal cold infusion**
- hot flashes

**Self-heal oil and cream**
- cuts
- sores
- wounds
- aches and pains
- swellings in the throat

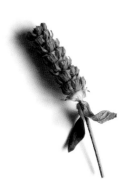

## Self-heal flower essence

To make the flower essence, find a patch of self-heal growing in a peaceful sunny spot. Just sit near the plants for a while until you feel relaxed and at peace with the plants and the place. Because flower essences are based on the vibrational energy of a plant rather than its chemistry, your intention is important.

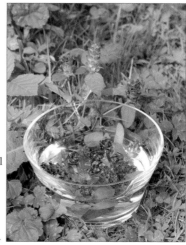

When you are ready, place a small clear glass bowl on the ground near the plants. Fill it with about a cupful of **rain water or spring water**, then pick enough **flowers** from nearby to cover the surface of the water. Leave them there for an hour or two – you can relax nearby or go for a walk while they infuse. The water will still look clear, but the flowers may have wilted. Use a twig to lift them carefully out of the water, and then pour the water into a bottle that is half full of **brandy.** This is called your mother essence. You can use any size of bottle you like, but a half pint blue glass bottle works well, and it may be easier to fill if you use a funnel. If there is any water left over, you can drink it.

**Flower essence**
- self-healing
- motivation
- inner direction
- transformation

To use your essence, put three drops of mother essence in a small (1 fl oz) dropper bottle filled with brandy. Using this stock bottle, you can:
- put 20 drops in the bath, then soak for at least twenty minutes.
- rub directly on the skin, or mix into creams.
- put a few drops in a glass or bottle of water and sip during the day.
- make a dosage bottle to carry around with you, by putting 3 drops of stock essence into a dropper bottle containing a 50/50 brandy and water mix or pure distilled rosewater. Use several drops directly under the tongue as often as you feel you need it, or at least twice daily.

Self-heal essence reminds us that all healing is self-healing, and is useful if you are ill and don't know where to turn for help. It will help you choose the therapies that will be beneficial, and enkindle your own innate healing energy. It can be used alongside any other form of treatment to enhance its effectiveness and benefits without any risk of negative interaction. Self-heal doesn't just work on a physical level, but will support the mental and emotional aspects of healing. It also helps to calm and center the spirit, benefiting meditation and prayer.

# Shepherd's purse *Capsella bursa-pastoris*

**Shepherd's purse stops bleeding of all sorts from nosebleeds to blood in the urine. It was used in First World War battles to staunch bleeding from wounds when ergot, an effective but more dangerous remedy, was not available.**

**Shepherd's purse also has an amazing ability to correct prolapses, especially of the uterus but also of the bladder, moving the organs back into their correct position.**

This common little herb, which most people know as a weed if at all, has an ancient history of herbal use, suggested in its beautiful Latin name. The plant's seed cases are said to resemble the heart-shaped satchels once worn on men's belts, whether shepherds or not.

### Use shepherd's purse for...

The aerial parts of shepherd's purse are all used herbally. Externally, it has been found excellent and safe in treating rheumatic aches and pains, and for ecchymosis, i.e., bleeding beneath the skin. Taken internally for kidney and bladder irritation, it is particularly good for mucus in the urine.

Less well known is its ability to treat prolapses. Julie had firsthand experience when she suffered a uterine prolapse. Within an hour of taking shepherd's purse tincture she could feel the uterus moving back into place, and three hours later the discomfort was mostly gone. She was back to normal in three days with the tincture, helped by yoga and reflexology.

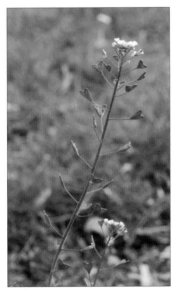

**Brassicaceae (Cruciferae) Cabbage family**

**Description:** Most easily recognized by its heart-shaped seed pods, this is a small annual with a rosette of slightly hairy, lobed leaves and tiny white flowers.

**Habitat:** Cultivated and disturbed ground.

**Distribution:** Native to Europe and Asia but widely naturalized in North America and other temperate regions.

**Parts used:** Above-ground parts.

Another case history involved a patient who had great discomfort and a bulging on the side of her vulva. She went to the nurse at the doctor's surgery, who examined her and said she had a uterine prolapse. The patient started taking shepherd's purse, and felt a fairly rapid improvement. Six days later,

**Contraindications**
Avoid taking shepherd's purse internally during pregnancy because it can stimulate uterine contractions.

**Fresh shepherd's purse plant**
- cuts
- nosebleeds
- rheumatism
- bleeding under skin

**Shepherd's purse tincture**
- bleeding
- heavy periods
- prolapses
- blood in urine
- wounds
- hemorrhoids

**Combined with hawthorn and lime blossom**
- high blood pressure

*Perhaps the most important cruciferous plant with medicinal use, it has been known as a haemostatic for centuries and evidence of its use has been found at Neolithic sites, probably as condiment and vegetable as much as medication.*
– Barker (2001)

her doctor examined her again and said the nurse must have made a mistake because the patient didn't have a prolapse at all.

Shepherd's purse also works for bladder prolapse. A woman had been diagnosed with this condition, which was causing her pain and discomfort. She didn't want surgery, so came to see Julie.

The patient took shepherd's purse and drank a bladder tea of uva ursi, couch grass, cornsilk, buchu, and horsetail. To support this, she began Pilates and did Kegel, i.e., pelvic floor, exercises. After a month she was greatly improved, and her doctor was amazed. Her urine had cleared. Two months later there were no signs of any problem and she felt fantastic.

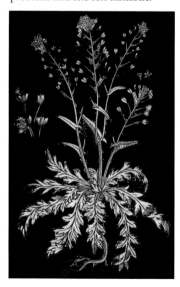

Illustration of shepherd's purse from *Theatrum Botanicum* by John Parkinson, published in 1640

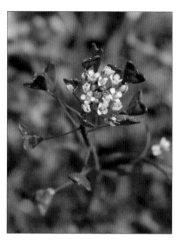

Shepherd's purse has small white flowers, which are quickly followed by the plant's signature heart-shaped pods.

Shepherd's purse has been used during childbirth to stimulate uterine contractions and reduce postpartum bleeding.

For high blood pressure, shepherd's purse combines well with hawthorn and lime blossom. Mix the tinctures together, using 5 parts hawthorn, 3 parts lime blossom and 2 parts shepherd's purse. Take 20 drops in a little water or juice twice a day.

During the First World War in Germany shepherd's purse was used as a less toxic substitute for ergot to stop bleeding. A case history to show its effectiveness for bleeding involves a man with blood in his urine. He went to his doctor for diagnosis, and found the blood was coming from weak blood vessels in his prostate. Shepherd's purse soon stopped the bleeding, and he then took bilberry to strengthen the blood vessels. He occasionally needed to take shepherd's purse over the next year, but had no later bleeding problem.

Shepherd's purse puts out flowers and seeds virtually all year round. It is best picked in the summer for making a tincture, but can be used fresh at any time. The leaves are tastiest before the flowers appear and can be eaten in salads; they are rich in vitamins A, B, and C. The seedpods can be used chopped up in soups and stews for their peppery taste. In Japan, shepherd's purse is grown as a vegetable and to flavor rice.

Because the flowering plant has a rather unpleasant taste, we prefer the tincture form (where a small dose is sufficient) rather than as an infusion or decoction, although these will work perfectly well too.

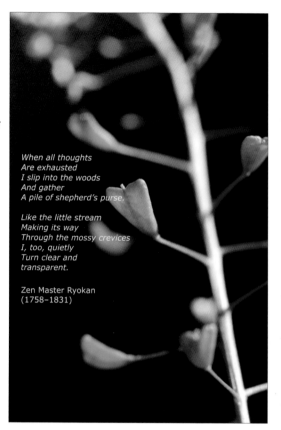

*When all thoughts*
*Are exhausted*
*I slip into the woods*
*And gather*
*A pile of shepherd's purse.*

*Like the little stream*
*Making its way*
*Through the mossy crevices*
*I, too, quietly*
*Turn clear and*
*transparent.*

Zen Master Ryokan
(1758–1831)

## Shepherd's purse tincture

Pick **shepherd's purse** while it is flowering, preferably in the summer. Fill a jar with the herb, then pour on **vodka** until it is covered. Put the jar away in a cool dark cupboard for a month, shaking the jar daily or as frequently as you can remember to do it. Strain off the liquid, pour it into a bottle and label.

**Dose:** For bleeding, take half a teaspoonful three times a day until the bleeding stops and then discontinue. For prolapse, 5 drops three times a day in a little water is usually sufficient. Continue taking it for a few days after everything has moved back into place.

## Formula for high blood pressure

Combine tinctures: 2 parts **shepherd's purse**, 3 parts **lime blossom** and 5 parts **hawthorn berry**.

**Dose:** 20 drops twice daily in water.

# St John's wort *Hypericum perforatum*

**St John's wort has become well known as an herb for treating depression and SAD, but it is far more than that. An antiseptic wound herb of ancient repute, it was the main plant of St John, the sun herb of midsummer and a protector against evil and unseen influences. In modern terms, it strengthens the nervous system and the digestion, protects the liver, is antiviral and reduces pain; it is a plant for support through life-cycle changes.**

**Clusiaceae (Hypericaceae) St John's wort family**

**Description:** A mid-sized perennial with yellow flowers. Distinguished from other species of *Hypericum* by the "perforations" in the leaf, which are actually oil glands.

**Habitat:** Roadsides, hedge banks, rough grassland, meadows, and open woodland.

**Distribution:** Native to Europe, an introduced weed in North America and Australasia.

**Related species:** There are several other species of St John's wort that look similar, but they are not as good medicinally, so check for the "perforations" in the leaf by holding one up to the sun.

**Parts used:** Flowering tops.

The protecting power of St John's wort derives from a powerful mix of observed herbal benefits and the plant's part in the Christian adaptation of older midsummer sun and fire "pagan" ceremonies.

Its Latin name *Hypericum* gives us clues about the takeover of one form of sun-magic by another. The *hyper-ikon* was an herb placed above St John's image, or painted icon; by extension, it meant power over ghosts or invisible bad spirits. It was particularly important to invoke the plant's help on St John's eve against witchcraft or diabolic influences (see panel on page 161).

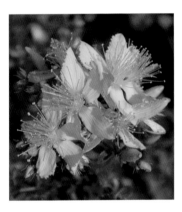

The cross formed by the leaves, seen from above, was also symbolic of the plant's power.

St John's wort was a powerful sun herb to dispel darkness, and it had the "signatures" to prove it. The so-called "holes" in the leaves, the *perforata* of the Latin name, were emblematic of St John's holy wounds and martyrdom, along with the red "blood" of the plant's extract. Scientists now know the holes to be resinous glands of hypericin and other active compounds.

The sun is said to control the solar (sun) plexus in the body. In yogic systems this is a center of protective energy that is ruled by the yellow part of the spectrum. This affinity of St John's wort with the solar plexus extends to the plant's use in treating the digestive and nervous systems. It is also taken for life-cycle conditions, such as bedwetting in the young, menstrual problems, and menopause. The solar plexus governs "gut instinct" and life's unseen influences – again leading us to protection.

This may sound rather esoteric, but we have certainly found for ourselves that the actual time of picking St John's wort flowers does matter in a practical sense.

We once gathered it on impulse on a summer evening while driving to a party in north Norfolk. We knew we should harvest in the middle of the day, but thought we'd try anyway. We put our beautiful yellow flowers into olive oil on arriving home, and placed the jar on a south-facing window-sill to infuse. Nothing happened. That jar was in the sun for months, but never turned red.

On the other hand, some of the best St John's wort oil we've ever made was on a visit to Italy. In Ostia Antica, the ancient harbor town for Rome, there were many interesting plants, including St John's wort, which was growing only among the ruined temples.

It was actually St John's day, June 24th, and very hot. We picked enough flowers to make a small jar of oil and infused it on our friend's balcony in Rome. Within hours it was a wonderful deep red color.

## Use St John's wort for...
What we find interesting is that modern uses of the plant, as we will outline, differ so much from

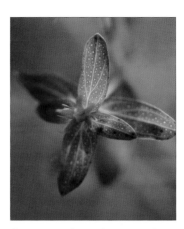

the more traditional uses. Look at Parkinson's list of its benefits (right): few herbalists will now use St John's wort to dissolve tumors. Mrs Grieve, writing in 1931, says it is good for pulmonary complaints, bladder problems, diarrhea, jaundice, and nervous depression, among others.

No mention there of a modern and effective use of St John's wort for what we now call seasonal affective disorder (SAD), where people feel low and depressed in the dark months of northern European winters. A spoonful of home-made St John's wort tincture will light you up inside with a warm glow.

St John's wort's reputation for helping lift the darkness of depression has grown considerably. This use of the herb has been well researched in the last twenty years and has stimulated a surge in sales of St John's wort products. It is known that hypericin interferes

When the light shines through the leaves of perforate St John's wort, the oil glands look like holes (hence *perforatum* in the name). There are ten times more glands in the flowers than the leaves or stems.

*S. Iohns wort is as singular a wound herbe as any other whatsoever, eyther for inward wounds, hurts or bruises, to be boyled in wine and drunke, or prepared into oyle or oyntment, bathe or lotion out-wardly... it hath power to open obstructions, to dissolve tumours, to consolidate or soder the lips of wounds, and to strengthen the parts that are weake and feeble.*
*– Parkinson (1640)*

**Caution:** Do not take St John's wort along-side antidepressant medication unless supervised by an herbal or medical practitioner. Seek professional advice before using the herb if you are on any medication, including the contraceptive pill, or are pregnant.

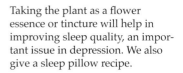

St John's wort growing along a Norfolk lane, St John's day, June 24th

with monoamine oxidase (MAO), which contributes to depression. Pharmaceutical products also act as MAO inhibitors, but St John's wort is a slow treatment, and, crucially, has few side effects.

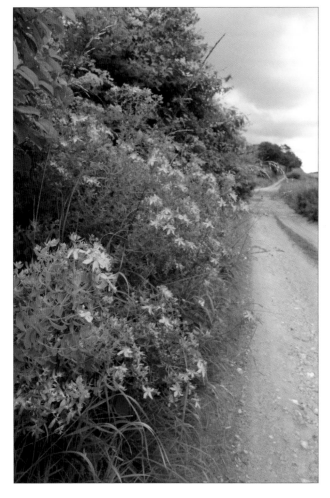

Taking the plant as a flower essence or tincture will help in improving sleep quality, an important issue in depression. We also give a sleep pillow recipe.

St John's wort treatment has been officially recognized in Germany since 1984 as effective for mild to moderate depression. When the protocol was publicized, St John's wort products soon outsold Prozac by a factor of seven to one.

A "modern" way of looking at depression has some interesting precursors. One example is an early nineteenth-century verse by Alfred Lear Huxford; this links a ceremonial use of St John's wort leaves bound to the forehead and the relief of "dark thoughts":

*So thus about her brow/ They bound* Hypericum, *whose potent leaves/ Have sovereign powers o'er all the sullen fits/ And cheerless fancies that besiege the mind;/ Banishing ever, to their native night/ Dark thoughts, and causing to spring up within/ The heart distress'd, a glow of gladdening hope,/ And rainbow visions of kind destiny.*

If you change the world-view from religious to scientific, from old "superstition" to modern "rationalism," is it really so far from fear of possession by evil spirits to modern clinical depression? Perhaps, like great literature, our major herbs adapt to the neuroses and psychic needs of the time; St John's wort has done this beautifully.

However, it would not be true to say the herb has no side effects at all. One, which is sometimes experienced among the fair-skinned, is to make them more sensitive to the sun. Care is needed if you burn easily, and the herb should be avoided if you need to be out in the sun and in danger of burning.

This proneness to sunburn extends to cattle. They are liable to gorge on the plant and can die, which is why many state laws have proscribed as noxious *H. perforatum,* the introduced St John's wort, also known as Klamath weed.

It was also an unwelcome chance arrival in Australasia and South Africa in the nineteenth century. Spreading by wind-borne seeds and active vegetative roots, it quickly overtakes native vegetation and local forms of the plant.

In the doctrine of signatures yellow-colored herbs are frequently associated with the liver and an ability to treat jaundice. This can be unfounded, but St John's wort is a case in point, working as it does to relieve liver tension and harmonizing the action of the liver with other digestive organs.

Its action is gently decongesting, strengthening both liver and gallbladder. But because St John's wort helps the liver break down and get rid of toxins, it can lower levels of certain drugs in the body, reducing their effectiveness. The best advice here is: do not use St

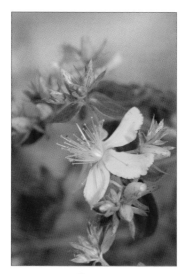

John's wort alongside any pharmaceutical medication without first seeking the advice of your herbal practitioner or doctor.

Taking St John's wort improves your absorption of nutrients, and helps normalize stomach acid levels whether too high or too low. It is a well-known treatment for ulcers, heartburn, and bloating.

It is also one of the best herbs for treating shingles, being antiviral as well as pain-relieving and also speeding up tissue repair. Use the infused oil externally over the painful area, and take the tincture internally at the same time.

As a proven antiviral, St John's wort may have future benefits for HIV and AIDS treatment, but more research is needed.

**Herbs of St John**
St John's wort is one of the main herbs of St John the Baptist, whose birthday was taken to be June 24th. It is no coincidence that John, the precursor of Christ, was given a birthdate in midsummer and Christ himself in midwinter. This was one way the year's solstices were appropriated from older pagan festivals by the Christian Church.

St John's wort, which blooms so brightly around midsummer, whether regarded as solstice or saint's day, is the name-plant for this time. Other herbs of St John were great plantain, mugwort, yarrow, and vervain (all in this book), and corn marigold, dwarf elder, ivy, and orpine (*Sedum telephium*).

The herbs of St John were gathered on the morning of June 23rd, before sunrise. That evening fires were lit, the smoke purifying both herbs and the people (and also cattle) who crossed the fires. The plants were now sanctified by the saint's power, and went into amulets, were placed above doorways and in cattle stalls, and stored for later use.

The overall protection afforded is well summarized in the French phrase *avoir toutes les herbes de la St-Jean,* meaning ready and safeguarded for everything.

**St John's wort tincture**
- seasonal affective disorder (SAD)
- mild depression
- liver congestion
- shingles
- nervous exhaustion
- menopausal moods
- viral infections
- jet lag

**St John's wort infused oil**
- backache
- sore muscles
- neuropathy
- neuralgia
- shingles
- arthritis
- surgical scars
- bruises
- sprains

**St John's wort pillow**
- nightmares
- bad dreams
- fear of the dark

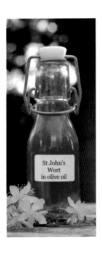

The oil also works well as a rub for backache and sore muscles and gums, and being antiseptic will help heal wounds arising from injuries or surgery, as in older formulations.

From its former reputation as a "cure-all" is derived the name of the garden St John's wort, tutsan, a corruption of the French name *La toute-sainte*.

### Harvesting St John's wort
St John's wort really needs to be picked on a sunny day, when the sun is high in the sky. Pick the **flowering tops** of the plant, i.e., the flowers, buds and leaves. The stems are quite wiry, so use a pair of scissors.

### St John's wort tincture
Put the **flowering tops** in a clear glass jar large enough to hold what you've picked, then pour on **vodka** until the herb is submerged. Put the lid on the jar, and shake to remove any air bubbles. Top up with a little more vodka if necessary.

Put the jar in a cupboard or other place away from the light for about a month, shaking occasionally. Your tincture is ready when the flowers have faded and the liquid is a reddish color. Strain, bottle, and label.

**Dose:** Half to one teaspoonful three times daily.

### St John's wort infused oil
Put the **flowering tops** you have picked into a clear glass jar, then pour on **extra virgin olive oil** until the herb is completely covered. Put the lid on and shake the jar to remove any air bubbles, then place on a sunny window sill for a month.

Check every now and then to make the sure the herb is still submerged in the oil, and if necessary stir it back under. The oil should turn red.

Strain off the oil, bottle, and label.

Use externally as needed for backache, sore muscles, sciatica, neuralgia, arthritic joints, and to help heal wounds.

### St John's wort pillow
Dry St John's wort flowering tops outside in the shade. Strip the leaves and flowers off the stalks and discard the stalks. Make a small cloth bag, leaving one end unstitched. Fill the bag loosely with the dried flowers and leaves, then stitch or tie the open end shut. Place the bag underneath your pillow.

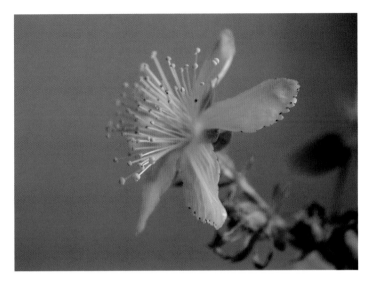

### St John's wort flower essence

Find a patch of St John's wort growing in a peaceful spot. On a clear sunny day sit near the plants for a while until you feel relaxed and at peace. Because flower essences are based on the vibrational energy of a plant rather than its chemistry, your intention is important.

Place a small clear glass bowl on the ground near the plants. Fill it with about a cupful of **rain water or spring water**, then use a pair of scissors to pick enough **flowers** to cover the surface of the water. Leave them there for an hour or two. The water will still look clear, but the flowers may have wilted. Use your scissors to lift them carefully out of the water, then pour the water into a bottle that is half full of **brandy**. This is your mother essence. You can use any size of bottle you like, but a half pint blue glass bottle works well, and it may be easier to fill if you use a funnel. If there is any water left over, drink it.

To use your essence, put 3 drops of mother essence in a small (1 fl oz) dropper bottle filled with brandy. Using this stock bottle, you can:
• put 20 drops in the bath, then soak for at least twenty minutes.
• rub directly on the skin, or mix into creams.
• put a few drops in a glass or bottle of water and sip during the day.
• make a dosage bottle by putting three drops of stock essence into a dropper bottle containing a 50/50 brandy and water mix. Use several drops directly under the tongue as needed, or at least twice daily.

**St John's wort flower essence**
• allergies
• environmental stress
• nightmares
• bedwetting
• seasonal affective disorder (SAD)
• protection

# Sweet cicely *Myrrhis odorata*

**Apiaceae
(Umbelliferae)
Carrot family**

**Description:** An aromatic perennial with foamy umbels of creamy white flowers, up to 3 ft tall.

**Habitat:** Stream banks, roadsides, grassy places, and gardens.

**Distribution:** A European plant that has been introduced to North America.

**Related species:** In North America, aniseroot or sweetroot (*Osmorhiza berteroi*) is also known as sweet-cicely. Both plants belong to a huge family, which includes many food plants but also a few poisonous species such as hemlock, so take care with identification.

**Parts used:** Leaves, flowers, unripe seeds.

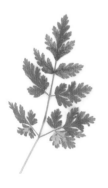

Sweet cicely is a common roadside plant in the dales of northern England, and is widely grown in gardens. The whole plant has a sweet aniseed flavor, giving it culinary uses. It is traditionally cooked with acid fruit, reducing the amount of sugar needed, and can be used as a sugar substitute by diabetics.

**Sweet cicely is an herbal tonic that restores energy, lifts the spirits and settles the digestion.**

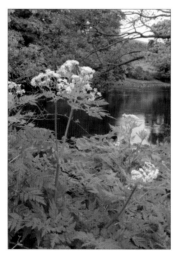

Like many herbs, sweet cicely was more widely used in the past than it is now. It was once valued as a protection against infection in the time of plague, and greatly appreciated in salads. Gerard, writing in 1597, said: "The seeds eaten as a sallad whiles they are yet green, with oile, vinegar, and pepper, exceed all other sallads by many degrees, both in pleasantnesse of taste, sweetnesse of smell, and wholsomnesse for the cold and feeble stomacke." He also liked the leaves in salads, and said that the boiled roots are not only tasty but very good for old people.

### Use sweet cicely for...
Sweet cicely still tastes just as good as it did all those years ago. It stimulates the appetite, relieves flatulence, griping and indigestion, and lifts the spirits. The whole plant is edible, and as Culpeper said: "It is so harmless, you cannot use it amiss."

Try the fresh young leaves, at their best before the plant flowers, chopped in salads. They can be used as a flavoring in cooking both sweet and savory dishes. Add the flowers to salads and desserts, or use as a garnish. The green unripe seeds can be nibbled to stimulate the appetite or to settle indigestion or gas and griping. They have a stronger flavor than the leaves or flowers. The young stems can be eaten too.

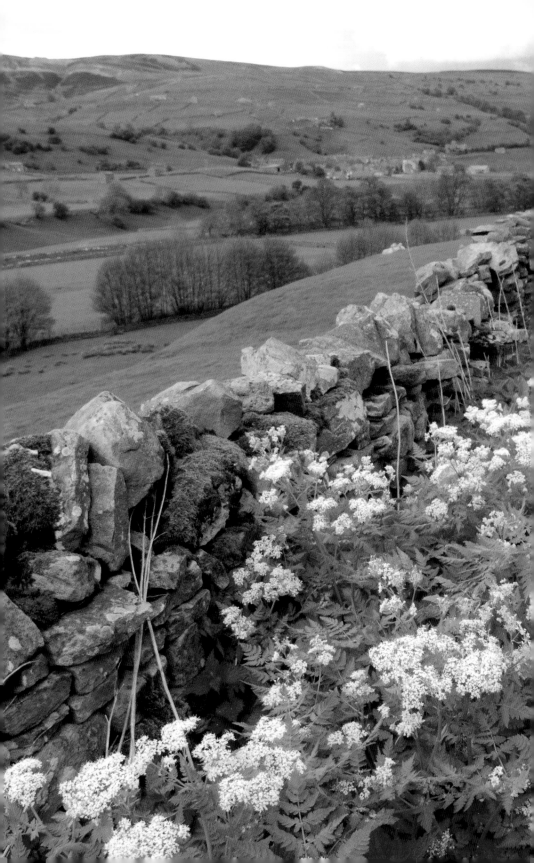

*Medicinally it has many virtues and few vices – so few that from the Greeks onward it was seen as a plant that could not be overused.*
*– Furnell (1985)*

Sweet cicely is particularly good for older people who have lost their enthusiasm for life, as it lifts the spirits and enkindles the digestive fire. It enables them to enjoy their food with good appetite, warming the digestion and improving absorption of nutrients.

This plant is also beneficial for anyone who is weak or exhausted, perhaps after a chronic illness or through caring for someone else. It will help them get back their energy and *joie de vivre*, slowly rebuilding their strength and gently warming the whole system.

**Sweet cicely apéritif**
• poor appetite
• weak digestion
• flatulence
• indigestion

### Sweet cicely apéritif

This can be drunk before meals to stimulate the appetite, or used as an after-dinner drink to settle the digestion. It can also be taken purely medicinally for flatulence, colic, or griping pains.

Use either a handful of green **sweet cicely seeds** or several handfuls of **leaves and stems.** Chop them up and put into a large, clean glass jar.

Add about a pint of **vodka**, and let steep in a dark place for two or three days. Taste it to check that the flavor of the herb has been absorbed by the alcohol, then strain and bottle in a clean glass bottle. The flavor improves if the bottle is left to age for two months in a dark place at room temperature before using.

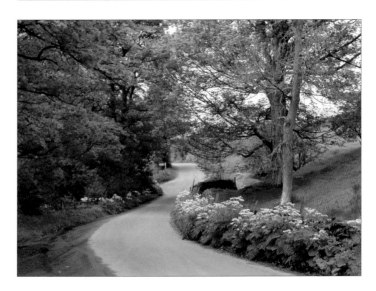

(*This and previous two pages*) Sweet cicely in the North Yorkshire dales, May

# Teasel *Dipsacus fullonum* syn. *D. sylvestris*

**Teasel is a stunning plant, tall and stately but also very beautiful if observed in detail when flowering. Its medicinal uses have long been appreciated in China, but are only recently being rediscovered by western herbalists.**

**Teasel helps with joint and tendon injuries, muscle pain and inflammation, chronic arthritis, and lower back weakness. It is now being used for Lyme disease, ME, and fibromyalgia.**

Teasel folklore has long referred to the way it collects rainwater in the cups where the leaves surround the stem, known from ancient times as the bath of Venus. This teasel water was said to be good for warts but particularly beneficial as an eyewash and as a wash for beautiful skin. We update this healing potential of teasel water with a home-made flower essence.

Teasel's famed commercial application is the use made of the dead flowerheads of the closely related fuller's teasel (*D. sativus*) in "teasing up" the nap on wool. *Taesan* is the Anglo-Saxon term for fulling or cleaning cloth. Common names for teasel like card weed, barber's brush, brushes, and gypsy's comb reflect this formerly important economic activity.

Fuller's teasel, with its hooked spines, was found to be uniquely effective both in manual and later in machine applications to raise the nap on fresh-made wool without breaking the cloth.

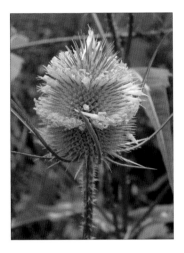

**Dipsacaceae
Teasel family**

**Description:** A tall biennial, up to 10 ft, with prickly rigid stems; small pale purple flowers in large conical flowerheads, opening from the middle; large and prickly basal leaves.

**Habitat:** Grassland, waste land, and by freeways.

**Distribution:** Native to Europe, introduced to North America.

**Related species:** This species is sometimes called fuller's teasel but the true fuller's teasel (*D. sativus*) has hooked spines that are used to card wool; Japanese teasel (*D. japonicus*) is used in Traditional Chinese Medicine.

**Parts used:** Root, flowers used as an essence.

## Use teasel for...

In Traditional Chinese Medicine, teasel root "tonifies the liver and kidneys" and works on painful lower backs and knees, weak legs, cartilage and joints. It is also held to promote circulation and reduce inflammation. American herbalists William LeSassier and Matthew Wood have built on these uses and found in practice that the teasel

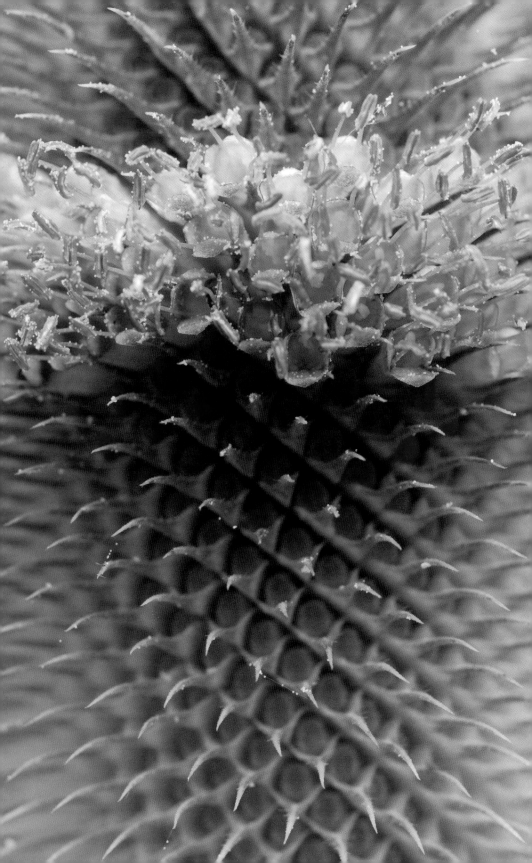

(introduced from Europe) is, in Wood's words, "invaluable" for joint injury and chronic inflammation of the muscles. It is indicated for fibromyalgia, chronic arthritis, and Lyme disease.

The acute infection of Lyme disease, as explained in an excellent monograph by herbalist Stephen Harrod Buhner (which any Lyme sufferer should buy), involves these same issues of joint pain, blood circulation, and tonifying of cartilage. Buhner finds results of using teasel root tincture for Lyme in the US are promising, though inconsistent in different regions.

Teasel flower essence has been found not only to bring relief in Lyme disease but also fibromy-algia, chronic fatigue, and lupus. Treatment for these complex conditions should be in consultation with an herbalist and your doctor.

Because teasel root has to be dug in the first year when the plant is harder to identify, and because using the root kills the plant, we prefer a recipe for a flower essence.

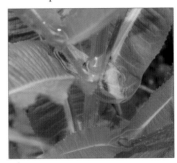

**Teasel essence**
Make this essence on a sunny day, using the **rainwater** collected for you by the teasel plant. Bend the plant over to pour some of the water from the leaf cups into a jug, then choose a flowerhead and bend it over into the jug so that it is immersed in the water for a minute or two. Alternatively, you can hold the flowerhead over a bowl and pour the rainwater from the jug over the blossoms into the bowl. If there is any debris in the water, filter it through a piece of muslin or a tea strainer as you pour it into a clean container to take home with you.

Measure the water and add an equal amount of **brandy** to preserve it. Bottle in a clean blue glass bottle, and label it.

To use, put three drops of this essence in a 1 fl oz dropper bottle filled with brandy. Add 20 drops to bathwater, or use as directed below.

**Dose:** Put 3 drops in a glass or bottle of water and drink during the day. Or put 3 drops into a small dropper bottle filled with half brandy and half water, and take by dropping a few drops directly under your tongue several times a day.

**Teasel essence**
• exhaustion
• chronic fatigue (ME)
• joint pain
• muscle aches

# Vervain *Verbena officinalis*

**Verbenaceae**
**Verbena family**

**Description:** A slender perennial, to 2 feet, with square stalks and spikes of small white or pale lilac flowers in late summer.

**Habitat:** Roadsides and grassy places, especially on dry soil.

**Distribution:** Found across Europe and Asia to Japan, and as an introduced species in many states in the US.

**Related species:** The North American blue vervain (*V. hastata*) can be used in place of vervain. Lemon verbena (*Aloysia triphylla*) is often called vervain.

**Parts used:** Above-ground parts when in flower.

**A prayer for picking vervain**
*All hail, thou holy herb, vervin,*
*Growing on the ground;*
*On the Mount of Calvary*
*There wast thou found;*
*Thou helpest many a grief,*
*And staunchest many a wound.*
*In the name of sweet Jesu,*
*I lift thee from the ground.*

An herb with a reputation for magic as well as medicine, vervain has a long history of use in Europe and Asia. It had so many reputed benefits that it gained a name as a cure-all; it was sacred for the Druids and used as an altar plant in ancient Rome.

It restores and calms the nervous system, is a digestive tonic and alleviates headaches. It is valuable for premenstrual tension, menopausal hot flashes, fevers, gallstones, jaundice, asthma, insomnia, anxiety, stress, and tension. Vervain is a wonderful restorative during convalescence from chronic or long-term illness.

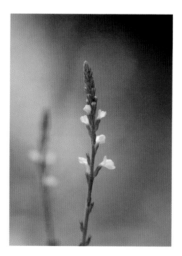

Vervain has a rich past, both magical and medicinal, sacred and secular. It was an important herb to the Druids and Romans. Picking was always accompanied, until recent times, by a prayer.

Once used to treat madness and epilepsy, vervain is a powerful nerve restorative, and is particularly good for nervous exhaustion following periods of prolonged physical activity or stress. It is excellent in convalescence for the weakness that follows viral infections. Julie has used it to treat ME/chronic fatigue syndrome.

Vervain is such a delicate plant that it is easy to overlook, but its medicinal power is belied by its humble appearance. Tincturing it is always surprising, as a few skinny stalks of pale lilac or white flowers yield a strong, dark, almost black, brew.

Vervain is a good herb to have on hand for the stress and hurried pace of modern lifestyles. It is particularly suited to people who are strong-willed, enthusiastic, work too hard, and cannot relax. It is one of Edward Bach's 38 original flower remedies, a specific for this type of intensity.

The physicians of Myddfai, in Wales in the thirteenth century, recommended vervain for scrofula, a tubercular infection of the lymph glands in the neck. Later, the great English herbalists had an uneasy relationship with the plant, Gerard decrying it and Culpeper favoring it. Parkinson (1640) chose the positive side by recommending vervain for "generally all the inward paines and torments of the body."

**Use vervain for...**
Because vervain works on the nervous system, liver, kidneys, and digestion and also balances hormones, in addition to being a wound herb, it is still valid in an unusual array of conditions, and deserves to be more widely used.

A vulnerary treatment in classical Rome, the crushed or chewed fresh leaf can still be applied to cuts and scrapes to soothe and promote healing. It is effective where there is heat and irritation, so works well on bramble scratches, boils, and burns.

Vervain had a role in both love and war in Rome. It was aphrodisiac, being dedicated to Venus: a Roman bride would wear a sprig at her wedding. A *verbenarius* was a herald-at-arms who wore a chaplet of vervain as a flag of truce.

Coming to recent times, research in the United States confirms that vervain, along with self-heal, is a top herb for normalizing levels

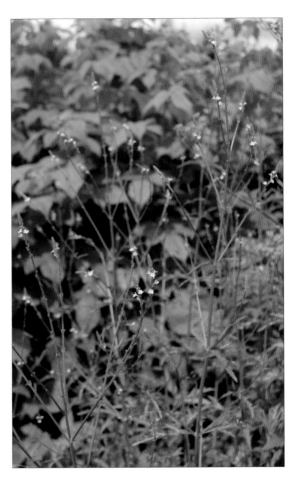

of thyroid hormones, being effective in both the underactive and overactive conditions. Vervain appears to affect the amount of TSH (thyroid-stimulating hormone) released by the pituitary gland.

Drinking vervain tea very hot will make you sweat, which means it is

*So many Virtues are attributed by Authors, to this Plant, that it would tire one to reckon them up.*
– Pechey (1707)

*Spenser called it 'vein-healing verven'. It had the old name of 'simpler's joy'.*
– Pratt (1857)

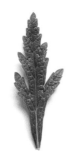

a really effective treatment at the start of a cold or fever, when you are actively eliminating toxins. But it also relaxes and soothes, settling an upset digestion as well as a preoccupied, racing mind.

As a tincture, vervain is cooling for menopausal hot flashes. It is particularly valuable to have available where restlessness and nervous tension are part of the menopausal picture.

Vervain tea is good for childhood illnesses, where the child is restless and irritable. Instead of fidgeting, he or she will be helped to relax and recuperate. If there is a fever, vervain will encourage

sweating and prevent the temperature from going too high. It combines well with lime blossom or elderflower for fevers.

Although there has been too little modern research on vervain, experience and the clinical practice of the herbalists who use it largely support its old reputation as a "heal-all." It is a safe remedy, gentle enough for children and convalescents, and tonic for older people.

Unfortunately, vervain seems to be becoming less common as a wild plant. If you can't find any near you, it is worth growing some in your garden for medicinal use. It self-seeds readily.

**Vervain tea**
- nervous tension
- anxiety
- colds and fevers
- premenstrual tension
- menstrual headaches
- poor absorption
- digestive problems
- inability to relax
- living on nerves
- hyperactivity
- thyroid imbalance
- muscular tension

**Vervain tincture**
- stress and tension
- anxiety
- premenstrual tension
- menstrual headaches
- nervous tension
- menopause
- hot flashes
- poor absorption
- digestive problems
- inability to relax
- living on nerves
- hyperactivity
- thyroid imbalance

### Harvesting vervain

Pick vervain when in flower, ideally toward the end of flowering. For use as a tea, dry the above-ground parts whole in a warm cupboard or in the open air on a piece of paper. When the plant is crisp, discard the larger stems and cut up or crumble into small pieces.

### Vervain tea

Use a heaped teasoonful of the **dried herb** per mug of **boiling water**, and allow to steep for 5 minutes. Strain and drink hot.

**Dose:** 1 mug three times a day. For insomnia from restlessness, drink a cupful or two in the evening. For sprains and deep bruises, 2 or 3 cups a day for at least three or four days.
**Combinations:** Mixes well with lime blossom for flavor and therapeutic value; also effective with self-heal.

### Vervain tincture

Chop up fresh **vervain** and put in a blender with enough **vodka** to cover. Blend briefly, then pour the mixture into jars and keep in a cool dark place for a week. Strain and bottle.

**Dose:** 20 drops in a little water three times daily.

# White deadnettle, Archangel

*Lamium album*

**White deadnettle is a uterine tonic with an ability to stop loss of fluids from the body, whether excessive menstrual flow, abnormal vaginal discharge, diarrhea, or a runny nose.**

**The leaves and flowers can be eaten, raw or cooked. The flowers are full of nectar, enjoyed by insects and children alike, and the leaves can be used as a poultice for cuts and splinters.**

The white deadnettle is so named because it resembles a stinging nettle, but has no stinging hairs. Other old names, such as deaf, dumb, or blind nettle, also refer to the plant's benign nature. The white deadnettle is also known as bee nettle, with stores of honey at the base of its corolla attracting the humble bees that fertilize it. The same sweet taste has also made sucking the white flowers irresistible to generations of children.

It can be confusing in spring when both the stinging and non-stinging plants, which often grow together, are in leaf and there are no flowers to distinguish them. The secret lies in the stem, which is square and hollow in white deadnettle, but round and solid in stinging nettle.

The white deadnettle is perhaps too common for its own good, and has been unduly neglected both as an attractive plant with some garden border potential – and making an excellent mulch – and for its many medicinal qualities.

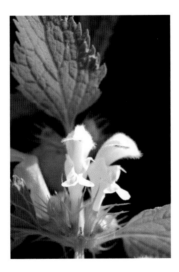

**Lamiaceae (Labiatae) Deadnettle family**

**Description:** Perennial with leaves similar to stinging nettle, but paler green and without the sting. Grows to 2 ft and has whorls of creamy white flowers.

**Habitat:** Roadsides, gardens, and waste ground.

**Distribution:** Found across north and central Europe to Asia; naturalized in North America and Australasia.

**Related species:** There are several other common species in the genus, but none that can be confused with white deadnettle. The other species were used medicinally in the past.

**Parts used:** Flowering tops whenever flowering, which can be at almost any time of year.

The plant's older name of archangel refers to Archangel Michael, whose day at one time correlated roughly with the first deadnettle flowers. We like the name for its protective connotations: the plant supports the female reproductive system and prevents the body from losing precious fluids through discharges of all sorts.

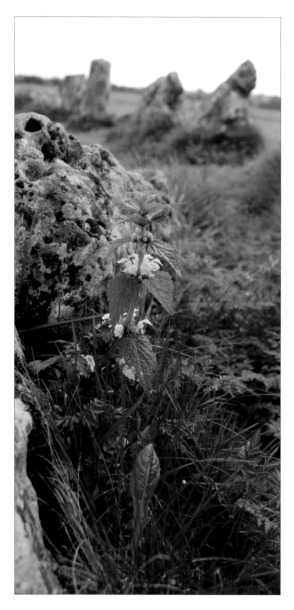

## Use white deadnettle for...

The main use herbalists make of the plant is as a uterine tonic. Julie finds it effective in treating painful periods and bleeding between periods, in reducing excessively heavy menstrual flow and for cystitis. It can be used for treating leucorrhea or vaginal discharge (once called "whites"), in which case the tea treatment (three cups a day) is continued for at least three weeks. A douche, made from a strong deadnettle tea, is good for vaginal discharges.

The tea also forms part of a treatment regime for benign prostate hyperplasia (BPH), and to speed recovery after prostate surgery.

The tea's mild astringency is supportive in treating respiratory complaints, especially where there is phlegm and catarrh.

White deadnettle also helps to regulate the bowel, and works well for gastrointestinal disorders, constipation, flatulence, and, in particular, diarrhea. It eases cramps and increases urination.

Externally, it has its uses in treatment as a poultice for cuts, bites, bruises, burns, splinters, varicose veins, and arthritic pain. For first aid, if you are out walking, the simplest method in the field is to chew deadnettle leaves and apply them to the sore point.

White deadnettle blooming at the Rollright Stones, Oxfordshire, April

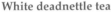

### Harvesting white deadnettle

White deadnettle can be found blooming almost any time of year, even right through the winter in mild areas. It is most prolific in the spring, but can be harvested whenever found in flower. Break off the stem a few leaves below the flower spikes.

If you want to store it, dry the sprigs whole, either by spreading them on a drying rack or paper, or by hanging small bunches tied with string or thread from the rafters or a laundry airer. When they turn crisp and dry, crumble the leaves and flowers, and discard stems.

### White deadnettle tea

Use a sprig of fresh flowering **white deadnettle**, or 1 to 2 teaspoons of the dried herb, per cup or mug of **boiling water**. Allow to infuse for about 10 minutes, then strain and drink.

**Dose:** 1 cup or mugful 3 times a day.

### White deadnettle douche

Make a strong tea with a handful of **fresh or dried herb** to 1 pint of **boiling water**, and let it infuse until cool. Strain, and inject the liquid into the vagina using a douche bag. Repeat once a day until the discharge stops. If it continues for a week, consult your doctor or herbal practitioner.

### Fresh white deadnettle leaf poultice

Pick the **fresh leaves** and either chew them or mash them with a mortar and pestle, then apply to the affected area and hold in place with a bandage or plaster. Change for a fresh poultice once or twice a day until healed, or, in the case of a splinter, until it is drawn out.

**White deadnettle tea**
- heavy menstruation
- painful periods
- vaginal discharge
- IBS
- cystitis
- diarrhea
- respiratory catarrh

**White deadnettle douche**
- vaginal discharge

**Fresh leaf poultice**
- burns
- bruises
- splinters
- cuts

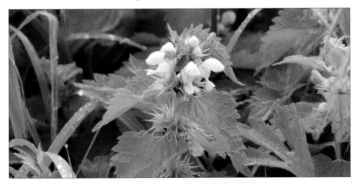

[the distilled water of deadnettle] *is used to make the heart merry, to make a good colour in the face, and to refresh the vitall spirits.*
– Gerard (1597)

*It is without question a gentle but really useful remedy for troubles of the reproductive organs in women, especially leucorrhoea.*
– Barker (2001)

# Wild lettuce *Lactuca virosa, L. serriola*

Asteraceae
(Compositae)
Daisy family

**Description:** Prickly lettuce *(Lactuca serriola)* is a 3–4 ft tall biennial with broad gray–green leaves and arrays of small, pale yellow flowers. Great (or greater) prickly lettuce, bitter lettuce, or lettuce opium (all *L. virosa*) is darker green, with purple, less spiny stems and similar small yellow flowers. Both species have distinctive spines along the underside of the midrib of the leaves.

**Habitat:** Roadsides, disturbed or waste ground.

**Distribution:** These two species are native to Europe, and introduced in North America. Prickly lettuce is generally more common than great lettuce.

**Related species:** Garden lettuce (*L. sativa*) can be used similarly, but is not as strong. Canadian lettuce (*L. canadensis*) is the most widespread North American wild lettuce.

**Parts used:** Leaves and latex, gathered when plant is in flower, in late summer.

**If you grew up with Beatrix Potter, you know from the** *Tale of the Flopsy Bunnies* **that eating flowering lettuces makes you sleepy. Our garden lettuces have been bred to reduce their bitterness, and as a result have far less of a soporific effect than does wild lettuce.**

The lettuce we buy in the shop or grow in our garden is a distant and hybridized relative of wild lettuce, but much altered in appearance and flavor. The only thing they have left in common is a milky sap or latex (*lactuca*) found in the stems of some commercial varieties and all through the plant in wilder varieties.

Strangely, though, if you allow a lettuce in your garden to "bolt" (i.e., flower and then seed), it reverts to something like the wild form, and recovers some of the healthy bitterness we try so hard to breed out of domesticated versions.

It is this bitter latex that is valued medicinally, and all lettuces have some of it. It is most abundant in great lettuce, less so in prickly lettuce and less again in garden forms. It can be harvested by cutting the flowering tops or leaves in summer and scraping off the juice. White when fresh, this juice oxidizes to brown in the air.

In this form it is known as lactucarium, and is chemically akin to opium, though unrelated botani-

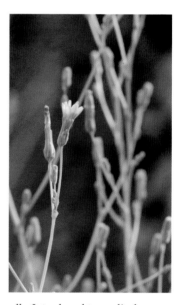

cally. Introduced to medical practice in 1771, it was later named lettuce opium. It was much used to adulterate opium in cough mixtures and as a sedative.

Lactucarium could be bought in British pharmacies until the 1930s and was still "official." Nowadays the only "official" part of wild lettuce is the dried leaves. It is just as well, lactucarium being unreliable in content and action.

Lettuce for insomnia is an old remedy. Galen, first-century AD physician to Roman emperor Marcus Aurelius, wrote: "I have found no better remedy for my trouble than eating lettuce of an evening."

But in one respect the reputation of lettuce has changed dramatically since ancient times. A form of cos lettuce, with its wild growth and white sap, was once held sacred to Min, the Egyptian god of fertility. But by the time of the ancient Greeks lettuce had become "the eunuch's plant."

Nowadays lettuce is a recognized anaphrodisiac, with a role in reducing sexual desire; externally, a cold lettuce tea is soothing and cooling for inflamed sexual organs. This effect works equally on both sexes (unlike hops). An old saying from Surrey went: "O'er much lettuce in the garden will stop a young wife's bearing."

Wild lettuce's sedative, cooling value extends to soothing the respiratory system, for dry, irritat-

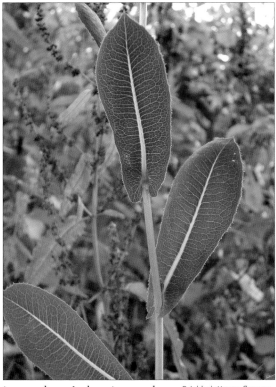

Prickly lettuce; flowers shown opposite

ing coughs and whooping cough. Relaxing spasm in the stomach and uterus, it relieves gripes and period pain. It is also beneficial for muscular and rheumatic pains.

---

**Wild lettuce tincture**

Harvest leaves and above-ground parts of wild lettuce while it is in flower in the summer. Take care of the spines. Chop it up and place in a blender with **vodka** to cover. Blend, then put the mixture into a jar and leave it in a cool dark place for two weeks. Strain and bottle.

**Dose:** Half a teaspoonful 3 times a day to calm over-excitement, or 1 teaspoonful at bedtime to help with sleep.

**Wild lettuce tincture**
• insomnia
• overactivity
• excitability
• colicky pains
• irritable coughs

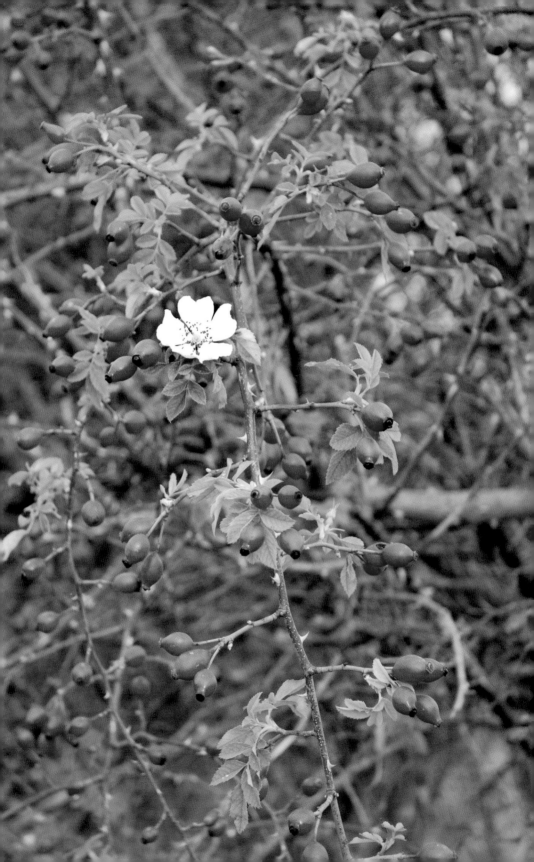

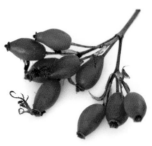

# Wild rose *Rosa* spp.

**For centuries the wild or dog rose was valued most for its galls, used to eliminate the stone. It wasn't until the 1930s that the hips became valued for their vitamin C, just in time for use in a rich syrup given to Britain's wartime children against infection.**

**Rose is the plant of love, the petals being the basis of the perfume industry. Herbally, it supports the immune system, is a good eliminator, and is cooling to the body.**

Autumn brings mist and mellow fruitfulness, in Keats's famous words, but he overlooks the frosts and flus of the fall. Fortunately, the fields and woods are "loaded and blessed" with a bounty of **rose hips** to help build up strength and resistance for the winter.

Everybody now knows that rose hips contain plentiful vitamins and minerals, but it was only in the 1930s that research established that home-grown hips had twenty, even forty times more vitamin C than oranges, plus good supplies of vitamins A, B, and K.

Oranges were to be an early casualty of the Second World War in Britain, and the Ministry of Food turned to the nation's school children to collect the domestic alternative. By 1945 amounts of 450 tons or so of rose hips were gathered each autumn to make into syrup; collectors were paid threepenny a pound, a useful bit of pin money for youthful entrepreneurs.

Rose hip syrup was rationed and provided to mothers for their children through the war years and for some time thereafter. The syrup (made by Delrosa) was in the shops, although Matthew, a post-war baby, remembers better the joy of seeing and eating his first orange in the early 1950s.

## Use wild rose for...
Rose hips and petals (the leaves are not used much) offer support to the body's immune system and help fight infection in the digestive tract; they are also diuretic, i.e., assist in elimination of wastes through the urinary system, as well as cooling to the body, bringing down fevers and reducing heat on the skin in the form of rashes and inflammations.

This threefold action – supporting immunity, helping elimination, and being cooling – makes rose a superb natural reliever of cold and flu symptoms, sore throats, runny noses, and blocked chests.

**Rosaceae**
**Rose family**

**Description:** Rambling deciduous shrubs with thorny stems and pink or white flowers, followed by bright scarlet hips in the fall.

**Habitat:** Field sides, scrub, and woods.

**Distribution:** Wild roses are found around the world, mainly in temperate areas.

**Species used:** There are many species, and they can all be used medicinally. Choose fragrant varieties if you are using the petals. Dog rose (*R. canina*) is the most common in Europe, with fragrant pale pink or white flowers and scarlet hips. North American native species include prickly rose (*Rosa acicularis*), prairie rose (*Rosa arkansana*), smooth rose (*Rosa blanda*), climbing rose (*Rosa setigera*), Virginia rose (*Rosa virginiana*), and Wood's rose (*Rosa woodsii*).

**Parts used:** Flowers gathered in midsummer and hips harvested in the fall

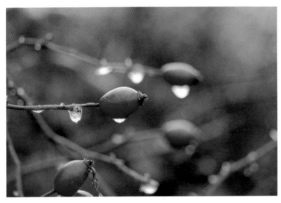

The effect is not only good for children, and rose hip tea as well as syrup are often given to convalescents and older people to improve their general resistance, as well as lighten their mood.

But there is one note of caution in this roll-call of autumnal virtue. The official wartime instructions emphasized that while the flesh of dog rose hips was so good for you the seeds, with their short hairs, were possibly dangerous if taken internally. However, the same hairs have provided "itching powder" fun for generations of boys.

Straining the stewed hips to remove the irritant hairs was specified in the recipe, and is still found in instructions for the syrup today.

**Rose petals** were favored by herbalists of old mainly for their cooling and astringent qualities, and to strengthen the heart and spirits. Today's herbalists use them in hormone-balancing formulae and for support in life-cycle stages. Rose hips, petals, and essential oil all buttress the nervous system, relieving insomnia, soothing the nerves, and lifting depression, as well as evening out heart palpitations and arrhythmias.

The astringent effect, particularly of the petals, is a result of high tannin levels, which help make rose useful in staunching bleeding and unwanted discharges. There is an effect too on the digestive system, cutting over-acidity and over-activity in the stomach, as well as reducing the spasms involved in diarrhea, colitis, and dysentery.

The petals have good antiviral properties and combine well with St John's wort, elder, and self-heal for treating viral infections. There are recent claims for good anti-HIV qualities in *R. damascena*, the damask rose.

Additionally, the petals, whether in the form of a water infusion, a distilled rose water or, as in our recipe, a glycerite, make a fragrant skin toner and cleanser, which will take the heat out of boils, acne, spots, and rashes. Rose water is also a soft, safe eyewash, mouthwash, and gargle, and a douche.

A story is told in *The Odyssey* of how good rose is for the skin, as well as winning the heart. Milto, a young girl and the daughter of a humble artisan, would put a fresh garland of roses each morning in the temple of Venus, the goddess of love. Milto was beautiful, but at one time a boil began to grow on her chin, and she became distraught.

In a dream the goddess came to Milto and told her to apply some of the roses to her face. She did so, and recovered her beauty and equanimity to such an extent that she later became the favorite wife of the Persian emperor Cyrus.

Rose petals make a wonderful cooling tonic for the whole female reproductive system, reducing uterine pain and the cramp of heavy periods, and supplementing other treatment of infertility and low libido. Rose's cooling and balancing qualities are particularly helpful during the menopause.

This is the ultimate feminine flower, found in practically every perfume, soap, and aphrodisiac, yet men often need it too, and rose can be used to treat impotence.

Rose has a softening action on the heart on an emotional level, and it is no accident that a dozen red roses are a conventional expression of the lover's feelings. Rose is prescribed by herbalists if the emotional aspect of "heart" is affected or there is a need for love. Rose helps us to love ourselves and be open to the love of others.

So, given all this, does the wild rose deserve its name "dog"? This might derive from derogatory

comments on its commonness – Pliny the Elder (AD 23–79), for example, thought Britain was named Albion because it was covered with white roses (*alba* meant white).

But rose's defenders prefer an origin from an Anglo-Saxon term meaning "dagger," for the thorn, or possibly the branch out of which dagger handles could be made. Another version of the name is that rose root was once thought to cure rabies, hence dog rose.

*Take three roses, white, pink and red. Wear them next to your heart for three days. Steep them in wine for three days more, then give to your lover. When he drinks, he will be yours forever.*
*– traditional love-charm, Germany*

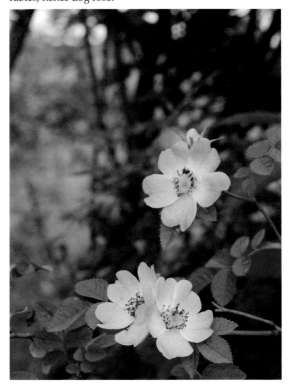

What may be less known today is that for centuries the main use of wild rose was for its gall or "briar balls," known as Robin's pincushions or bedeguars. Apothecaries ground them into a powder and sold them to treat kidney or bladder stone and as a diuretic. This use is long obsolete.

In any event, the success of the modern domesticated rose owes much to the wild form, and it is still usual for more tender species of ornamental roses to be grafted on to a wild rootstock. The petals of your garden roses can be used medicinally, if they are fragrant.

The Seals have a family story of rose grafting. Matthew's grandfather Ted Seal lived in Leicester and was a fervent gardener. For a private joke he grafted some big blowsy roses on to wild briars growing by the railway line to London.

He said he wanted to confuse the passengers and make them think the country roses near Leicester were something special. Perhaps he was one of those people who knew that thorns have roses.

**Rose petal glycerite**
- viral infections
- hormone balance
- menopause
- dry skin
- feeling unloved
- feeling unloving
- grief
- loneliness

### Rose petal glycerite

You can use garden roses along with wild roses for this recipe, as long as they haven't been sprayed.

Pick fragrant **rose petals** and put them in a jar with a mixture of 60% **vegetable glycerine** and 40% **water**. Put the jar on a sunny window ledge or in a warm place. Stir occasionally to keep the petals beneath the surface of the liquid. You can add more petals over the season, removing any that have turned transparent. When the last petals have lost their color, strain off the liquid and bottle. It should have a powerful aroma of rose, and taste heavenly.

**Uses**: 1 teaspoonful as needed for sore throats or viral infections.
For a "broken heart" or grief, mix half and half with hawthorn tincture and take 1 teaspoonful several times a day. Rose glycerite is a pleasant addition to many herbal tinctures and formulae.
As a face lotion for dry or delicate skin, mix half and half with water and apply daily.

### Rose hip vinegar

Put 20 or 30 **rose hips** in a jar or flask and cover with **apple cider vinegar**. If you want to speed up the process, slit the skins of the hips with a sharp knife before putting them in the vinegar. Leave on a sunny window sill for about a month, then strain and bottle.

**Uses:** For sore throats, mix a tablespoonful with a little warm water, gargle, and then swallow. For colds, make a drink using a tablespoon of rose hip vinegar in a mug of hot water, sweetened to taste with honey; or use in salad dressings.

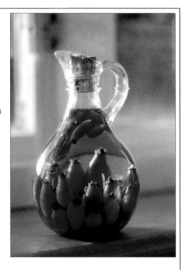

**Rose hip vinegar**
- colds
- sore throats
- salad dressings

**Rose hip syrup**
- colds
- sore throats
- source of vitamin C

### Raw rose hip syrup

Gently score a few lines through the skin of red **rose hips**, then layer them in a wide-mouthed jar with enough **sugar** to fill up all the gaps between the hips. Leave on a sunny window sill for a couple of months or until the sugar has drawn the juice from the hips and liquified. Strain off the liquid, bottle, and store in the fridge. This is a really thick and delicious syrup. Take a teaspoonful or two daily to prevent colds.

### Boiled rose hip syrup

This is the more traditional way to make the syrup, and what it may lose in vitamin C content it gains in having a longer shelf life.

Measure the volume of the **rose hips** you have picked, then pour them into a saucepan with half their volume of **water** (1 pint water to 2 pints hips). Boil hips and water for 20 minutes in a covered saucepan. Allow to cool, then strain through a jelly bag. For every 2 cups of juice, add 1 cup **sugar**. Boil for 10 minutes and pour while still hot into sterilized bottles. Label bottles when cool. Take a teaspoonful or two daily to prevent colds, or more frequently as needed for sore throats and colds.

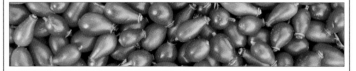

*In Wynter and in Somer it [Syrope of Rooses] maye be geuen competently to feble sicke melacoly and colorike people.*
– Askham's Herbal (1550)

# Willow *Salix alba, S. fragilis, S. nigra*

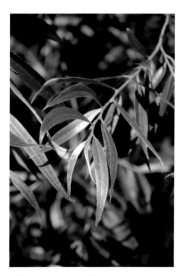

**Willow bark contains salicin and other aspirin-like compounds. It is used to treat pain and inflammation, but does not have the stomach-irritating or blood-thinning effects of aspirin.**

**Willow helps to lower fevers, and can be used as a gentle pain reliever for headaches, arthritis, gout, rheumatism, muscle aches, and lower back pain.**

**Salicaceae
Willow family**

**Description:** Tall deciduous trees that frequently hybridize with each other.

**Habitat:** Mainly riverbanks and other wet areas.

**Distribution:** Willows are found all around the world, in a wide variety of habitats.

**Species used:** Crack willow (*S. fragilis*) usually has higher levels of salicin than white willow (*S. alba*), which is the species mentioned in most herbals.
In North America, the black willow (*S. nigra*) is the main species used. Many species are used medicinally worldwide.

**Parts used:** Bark, collected in spring, and leaves.

*It is a fine cool tree, the boughs of which are very convenient to be placed in the chamber of one sick of a fever.*
– Culpeper (1653)

*The branch tips and leaves, known as willow tips... are traditionally used in many parts of South Africa to treat rheumatism and fever.*
– Van Wyk et al. (1997)

Willows are graceful trees often found growing by water. White willow is particularly elegant, with its silvery leaves swaying in the wind. Crack willow is so named because the fast-growing trunk often cracks and splits under its own weight. The familiar silver catkins, "pussy willow," are from the sallows, a group of willows with broader leaves.

Willows are highly adaptable trees, and will usually root readily from a stick put in the ground. Willow leaves, mashed up and soaked in water, can be used as a natural rooting hormone to help root cuttings of other plants.

Willows have many uses. The flexible shoots, mainly of osier (*Salix viminalis*), make excellent wicker baskets, and the wood of a variety of white willow is used commercially for clogs and cricket bats. Willow wood is burnt to make charcoal for drawing, and willow charcoal was once used in producing gunpowder.

Willow contains high levels of pain-relieving salicin. The modern use of aspirin is said to begin in 1763 when Rev. Edmund Stone extracted salicylic acid from willow bark for his parishioners' use. During the nineteenth century various scientists produced salicylic acid in the laboratory, and in 1853 the French chemist Charles

Gerhardt made a primitive form of aspirin. Later a German chemist discovered a better method for synthesizing the drug, and it started being marketed by Bayer in 1899. Aspirin, acetylsalicylic acid, is one of the most widely used drugs in the world today.

Interestingly, the early herbals do not focus on willow for relieving pain but more on its astringent action in stopping bleeding, diarrhea, and other "fluxes." The leaves, boiled in wine and drunk over an extended period of time, were considered an effective treatment to reduce lust in both sexes.

It is possible that willow was used for pain as a folk remedy that didn't make it into the books. Willow bark was chewed by country folk to relieve headaches and toothache, and to treat the ague, a type of malarial fever.

Today herbalists use willow mainly for pain, inflammation, and fever. Our son, who suffered from ME for several years as a young

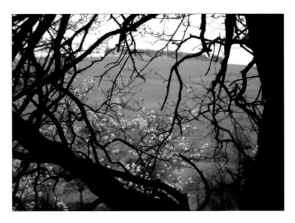

teenager, always asked for it for his headaches and muscle aches and pains. Like meadowsweet, it is effective for arthritis and rheumatism, and can help with the pain of polymyalgia rheumatica and fibromyalgia, for which it combines well with Guelder rose.

Note that if you are taking aspirin as a blood thinner, you cannot replace it with willow, which lacks this effect. But for long-term pain relief willow may be better for the stomach than aspirin.

Pussy willow, Shropshire, in April.

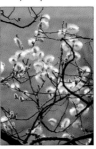

**Cautions:** Do not take willow if you are allergic to aspirin or while breastfeeding.

**Willow bark tincture**
- aches and pains
- headache
- arthritis
- rheumatism
- muscle aches
- backache
- gout
- period pain
- colds and flu
- sports injuries

**Willow bark tincture**
Harvest the bark in the spring, from branches where it isn't too thick. Use a sharp knife to strip thin slices of bark lengthwise off the branch on one side, taking care not to take too much from any one place.

Put the **willow bark** in a jar, and pour in enough **vodka** to cover it. Leave it in a cool dark place for a month, shaking regularly every few days. Strain off the liquid, bottle, and label it.

**Dose:** 1 teaspoon three times a day, taken in a little water when needed for relief of pain and inflammation.

# Willowherb *Epilobium* spp.

**Onagraceae**
**Willowherb family**

**Description:** Perennials growing up to about 2 ft, recognizable by small pink flowers, which have four notched petals, borne on the ends of long seed-pods. These split and curl when ripe to release downy seeds.

**Habitat:** Gardens and other disturbed ground, woods and damp places.

**Distribution:** Widespread throughout the northern hemisphere.

**Species:** There are about ten species, which are used interchangeably, including American or fringed willowherb (*E. ciliatum*), marsh willowherb (*E. palustre*), hoary or smallflower hairy willowherb (*E. parviflorum*), and broad-leaved willowherb (*E. montanum*).

**Related species:** Rosebay willowherb has been reclassified into the genus *Chamerion*, but is closely related. The great willowherb, also known as codlins and cream (*E. hirsutum*), is not used in herbal medicine – it grows to 5 ft, has large cerise flowers, and grows in ditches or by streams.

**Parts used:** Above-ground parts in flower.

**The small-flowered willowherbs are a specific remedy for prostate problems, including benign prostate hyperplasia (BHP). Plants in this informal group help shrink the tissues, arrest cell proliferation, and normalize urinary function.**

**Small-flowered willowherbs are also effective for a wide range of bladder and urinary problems, for women as well as men, with the astringent and diuretic action serving to tone and also detoxify the urinary tract.**

The Austrian herbalist Maria Treben was the first to bring the small-flowered willowherbs to public attention in recent times. She wrote of helping hundreds of people with prostate problems by using this neglected herb.

Julie's father, living in Namibia (which still has a strong German influence from colonial days), drank willowherb tea for his prostate twenty-five years ago, but the tea is still not widely available for sale in the UK. All the more reason to grow or pick your own!

These willowherbs frequently appear as garden weeds because they like bare or disturbed soil. If you break the stem about halfway up, the plant will grow new side shoots, and you can collect from the same plant several times during the summer.

Any of the small-flowered species can be used (see panel on the left), which is handy because they

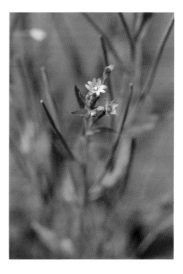

hybridize easily and are difficult to identify individually. The flowers vary in color from deep pink almost to white, and leaf shapes range from very narrow to quite broad, and from smooth to downy.

The name willowherb comes from the willow-like leaves. The flowers of some species look like burning matches, with the bright pink buds at the end of long ovaries or unripe seed pods (or cods as the old English herbalists call them).

These writers classified willow-herbs with the loosestrifes. Gerard describes the seed "wrapped in a cottony or downy wooll, which is carried away with the winde when the seed is ripe," but apparently didn't use the plant. Parkinson calls it very astringent and "effec-tuall both to stanch blood, restrain fluxes, heale the sores of the mouth and secret parts, close up quickly greene wounds and heale old ulcers."

While best known as a prostate remedy, these plants aren't just for men. They can help women with bladder and urinary problems too, used on their own or with pellitory of the wall, couch grass, horsetail, and bilberry leaves. For prostate enlargement, willow-

herbs can be taken alongside nettle root, another effective remedy for the condition. But do consult your herbalist or doctor first.

It is well worth keeping a little patch of willowherbs in a corner of your garden. They are persistent, growing up in cracks or unweeded bare soil, so once established you'll have a ready supply on hand (we know gardeners will regard these words as heretical).

*Everyone who knows this herb values and preserves it through careful picking.*
– Treben (1983)

These two specimens from our garden show how variable in form small-flowered willow-herbs can be in even a small area

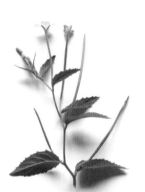

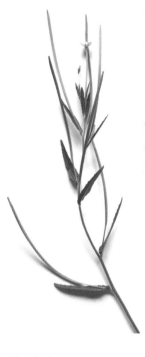

### Harvesting willowherb
Harvest by picking the flowering stems about halfway up. This enables the plant to produce more flowers and seeds later on. Dry in a shady place. As the plants dry, the seed pods often break open and release tiny downy seeds, so you might want to do this outdoors. You can use the whole plant, but the tea is more manageable if you discard the fluffy seeds and larger stems, then cut into small pieces with a pair of scissors and store in jars or brown paper bags in a cool dry place.

### Willowherb tea
Use a heaped teaspoonful of the **dried herb** per mug of **boiling water**, and infuse for about 3 minutes. Drink two to three cups a day. Maria Treben recommends 1 cup in the morning on an empty stomach and another half an hour before the evening meal.

**Willowherb tea**
• prostate enlargement
• urinary problems
• bladder disorders
• diarrhea

# Wood betony Stachys officinalis syn. Betonica officinalis

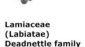

**Lamiaceae
(Labiatae)
Deadnettle family**

**Description:** A perennial up to 18" tall, with bluntly toothed leaves in a rosette, and bright magenta flowers.

**Habitat:** Heaths, woodland clearings, grassy places, and gardens.

**Distribution:** Naturalized in Massachusetts and New York state, native to Europe.

**Related species:** Other *Stachys* species include woundworts and hedgenettles.

**Identification:** Wood betony is easily distinguished from its relatives by its bluntly toothed leaves.

**Parts used:** Leaves and flowers.

**Wood betony, often referred to simply as betony, was a significant remedy from ancient times. A Roman physician wrote a whole book extolling its virtues, and it was the herb of choice for exorcising demons and protection against all kinds of evil in the Middle Ages.**

**Wood betony is a nerve tonic, and through its action on the solar plexus has a wide range of benefits, especially on the digestion. It also improves circulation, and is excellent for the elderly.**

Wood betony is another herb that does so much that it is hard to know where to start in writing about it. It is a pretty, orchid-like but easily overlooked plant, and, appropriately, works quietly to improve health over a broad front.

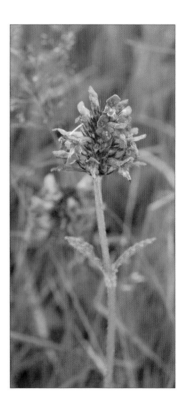

As an herbal all-rounder it was well known to the ancients. Culpeper (1653) relates that Antonius Musa, physician to Emperor Augustus, wrote a monograph on it, listing 47 different disorders betony would cure, among them protection from snakes and evil.

Anne Pratt, writing in the mid-nineteenth century, notes that betony was still highly valued in Italy. She quotes two current proverbs: "May you have more virtues than betony," as a farewell to a friend, and "Sell your coat, and buy betony," for those in pain.

Parkinson (1640) sums up the reputation of betony in his own day, neatly indicating the link he valued of "daily experience" and the authority of the ancients:

*It is found by daily experience, as Dioscorides formerly wrote thereof, to be good for innumerable diseases.*

Betony was venerated by the Celts, and its common name is thought to be a corruption of two Celtic words: "bew" for head, and "ton" for improve, making clear its power to cure head problems.

Throughout the Middle Ages this was an herb cultivated in monastic gardens and graveyards, for protection against witchcraft. Amulets of betony would be worn around the neck or placed under the pillow for personal protection.

It could be that betony's old reputation as a protector stems from its ability to help us face the fears and evils in our own minds. The *Grete Herball* (1526) made sure by combining a betony remedy with wine "for them that ben to ferfull:"

*gyue two dragmes of powdre hereof wt warme water and as moche wyne at the tyme that the fere cometh.*

### Use wood betony for...
Perhaps this echo of magic and folklore has swayed many classically trained herbalists against betony, and some modern writers are dismissive of its efficacy. We see it as an herb, like St John's wort or vervain, that meets ever-changing physical and spiritual needs.

Today it is best known as a nerve tonic, which strengthens the entire nervous system. Betony calms and relaxes, helping release stress and tension from both mind and body.

It is an excellent herb for insomnia stemming from nervous tension, where endless thoughts keep churning and you just can't let go and relax. Have a cup of the tea or a few drops of the tincture in the evening for deep relaxation, followed by a restorative sleep.

Betony was once used to treat madness, and can still have a useful role in some psychiatric disorders. Herbalists favor it for people coming off addictive drugs or recovering from head injuries.

Betony is beneficial for several kinds of headache, including tension, migraine, and liverish types. It helps when there is a feeling of spaciness and unconnectedness as well as in cases of frantic mental activity and scattered thoughts.

Because betony affects the solar plexus, it assists in a wide range of digestive problems, harmonizing the action of the entire digestive tract. It is helpful both when anxiety, irritability, or depression are affecting the digestion, or digestive upsets are upsetting the mind.

Betony stimulates a weak digestive tract but also soothes and calms it. It is helpful when there is irritable bowel syndrome, gastritis, colitis, and other conditions

*We have often seen in cottages in Kent... large bundles of the 'medicinal Betony', as Clare calls it, hung up for winter use.*
*– Pratt (1857)*

*Thy wild-woad on each road we see;*
*And medicinal betony,*
*By thy woodside-railing, reeves*
*With antique mullein's flannel-leaves.*
*– Clare, 'Cowper Green' (1828)*

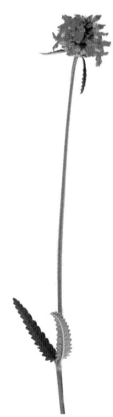

with inflammation and tension in the gut. It is the perfect remedy for "butterflies in the stomach" and for reconnecting us to "gut instincts." When we are "too much in our heads," it can bring us down to earth, to a more grounded level of reaction and feeling.

Betony also improves concentration and memory, which, combined with its calming qualities, makes it a good choice during examinations or other stressful times in our lives when we need to be able to focus and concentrate.

With effects on memory, circulation and digestion, betony is an ideal herb for older people or anyone recovering from long-term illness. It will gently warm and invigorate the whole system, increasing mental and physical strength. It improves the appetite and supports those who are too thin in regaining healthy weight.

Betony increases tone throughout the body, so can assist with prolapses of the uterus and other organs. It is used for weak labor, excessive menstrual bleeding, poor respiration, debility, and liver and gallbladder problems.

Like self-heal, wood betony is a good choice for when you don't quite feel well but don't really know what the problem is.

Wood betony growing in a meadow in Lincolnshire, June

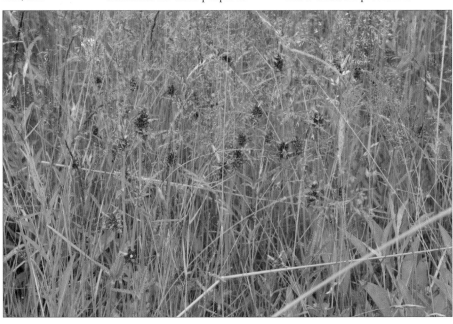

## Harvesting wood betony
Pick the plant just before the flowers fully open. To dry for a tea or pillow, spread on a screen or brown paper in the sun. When dry and crisp, put into brown paper bags or jars to store.

## Wood betony tea
Use 2 teaspoonfuls of the fresh herb or 1 teaspoonful of the dried herb per cup of boiling water, and leave to infuse for 10 to 15 minutes.

**Dose:** 3 cups a day, or 1 cup at bedtime to relax for a good night's sleep.

## Wood betony tincture
Put fresh **wood betony herb** in a blender with enough **vodka or brandy** to cover. Blend briefly, then pour into a jar and put in a cool dark place for a week. Strain off the liquid, bottle, and label.

**Dose:** Wood betony often works very well in drop doses. Take 5–10 drops in a little water three times a day. For insomnia, take 10 drops at bedtime. For more of a tonic effect, take 1 teaspoonful three times a day.

## Wood betony ointment
Pick a handful of **wood betony leaves**, chop them, and put in a small saucepan with half a cup of **extra virgin olive oil**. Using a low heat, warm gently, just below simmering, until the leaves have lost their green color and are quite crisp. Strain, returning the oil to the pan.

Add half an ounce of **beeswax** and warm until it melts. Stir well and pour into jars. Leave the lids off until the ointment sets, then label and store in a cool place until needed.

## Wood betony pillow
Sew a small cloth bag, leaving one end open. Fill loosely with dried wood betony leaves. Some dried lavender flowers or rose petals can be added for their fragrance. Stitch or tie up the open end, and place the bag under your pillow.

## Wood betony, hawthorn and horseradish formula
Mix 5 parts **wood betony tincture**, 4 parts **hawthorn tincture or syrup** and 1 part of **horseradish vinegar**. This formula stimulates and warms, improving digestion, circulation, and memory.

**Dose:** 1 teaspoon morning and afternoon as a tonic for older people or anyone recovering from a long illness. Also great for exam time!

**Wood betony tea**
- insomnia
- digestive problems
- headache
- poor circulation
- low appetite
- muscular tension
- nightmares
- sinus congestion
- watery, irritated eyes
- head colds
- chills and fevers

**Wood betony tincture**
- headache
- feeling of spaciness
- digestive problems
- vertigo
- memory loss
- nervous exhaustion
- anxiety
- irritability
- poor concentration

**Wood betony ointment**
- bruises
- sprains
- strains
- varicose veins
- hemorrhoids

**Wood betony pillow**
- insomnia
- nightmares

**Wood betony, hawthorn, and horseradish formula**
- tonic for older people
- convalescence
- exams

**Caution:** Do not take during pregnancy.

# Yarrow *Achillea millefolium*

**Asteraceae
(Compositae)
Daisy family**

**Description:** A short perennial with feathery dark green leaves and flat heads of white or sometimes pink flowers.

**Habitat:** Roadsides, meadows, and lawns.

**Distribution:** Found virtually worldwide.

**Related species:** Several species of *Achillea* are used medicinally and others are grown as garden plants.

**Parts used:** Above-ground parts collected when flowering, or leaves gathered as needed.

Yarrow or milfoil is a leading backyard medicine plant. A ready first-aid treatment for wounds and nosebleeds, it has larger uses as a circulatory system remedy that both stops bleeding and moves stagnant blood, preventing and clearing blood clots. It tones the blood vessels and lowers high blood pressure.

Yarrow is beneficial for a wide range of menstrual problems, and is a first-rate fever herb, used as a hot tea to induce sweating.

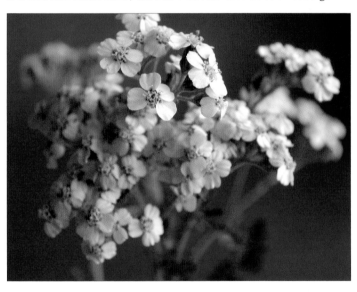

**Cautions:** Yarrow can occasionally cause an allergic skin irritation. It is best not given to children under 5 years old, or taken by pregnant or breastfeeding women.

Yarrow is a famous wound and fever herb, yet today it can pass unnoticed except as a lawn weed. The legendary Achilles used yarrow as a field dressing for his soldiers' wounds in the Trojan war, and the plant is named for him. A pity, then, he had none handy for his own fatal heel wound!

**Use yarrow for...**
Yarrow is our favorite remedy for nosebleeds, and it's well worth keeping a patch by the back door if anyone in your family suffers from them. Simply pick a few fresh leaves – available year round, though at their best in spring and the fall – and rub them

between your hands to bruise them, releasing the aromatic oil. Roll the leaves into a nasal plug, insert into the affected nostril and leave until the bleeding completely stops before gently removing the plug.

Julie's father suffered a really bad nosebleed once in the middle of the night, but luckily we had a patch of yarrow close by and the bleeding was soon stopped.

Yarrow has a traditional reputation of being able to start a nosebleed as well as stop one, from a time when bleeding was considered desirable as a cure for migraine. Indeed, one of the plant's old names was "nosebleed."

It is certainly as effective at breaking up congealed blood as it is at stopping hemorrhages, making it a valuable first-aid remedy for thrombosis, for blood blisters and bruises with bleeding beneath the skin, as well as hemorrhoids. If treating for hemorrhoids, take yarrow tea or tincture internally, and place a yarrow poultice or compress over the affected area.

This special ability to both stop bleeding and break up stagnant blood makes yarrow a valuable menstrual remedy. It will correct both heavy and suppressed periods, and will normalize blood flow if there is clotting.

It is also a remedy for vaginal discharge and helps prevent painful periods. Austrian herbalist Maria Treben considered yarrow "first and foremost a herb for women."

This has truth, but the plant's old names of soldier's woundwort and knight's milfoil bring us back once more to yarrow's affinity for battlefields and for being a wound-packing material, probably long before the Achilles myth was recorded. Its use paralleled the development of weapons, and it was the *herba militaris*, the herb dressing carried by battle surgeons around the world until at least the American Civil War.

Yarrow has long had a particular repute for closing bleeding wounds caused by weapons or tools made of iron. In France it is called the *herbe au charpentier* (English version: carpenter's grass) for the same reason. It is useful to know in case of domestic or outdoor accidents that yarrow's emergency help can be at hand. Find a plant, strip the leaves, crush them and pack into the wound: it is antibacterial and antimicrobial so you will not introduce infection.

The reason why yarrow is so versatile – it was known as a "cure-all" herb – is that it works to tone the blood vessels, especially the smaller veins, and lower blood pressure by dilating the capillaries. This means it has a beneficial whole-body effect through the blood system, especially on conditions related to hypertension and including coronary thrombosis.

*Yarrow has proved beneficial in the treatment of so many illnesses and afflictions that no garden should be without it.*
– Roberts (1983)

*Achillea is an important diaphoretic herb, and is a standard remedy for helping the body deal with fever. It stimulates digestion and tones blood vessels.*
– Hoffmann (2003)

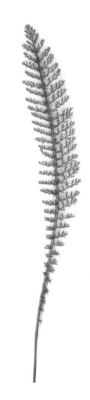

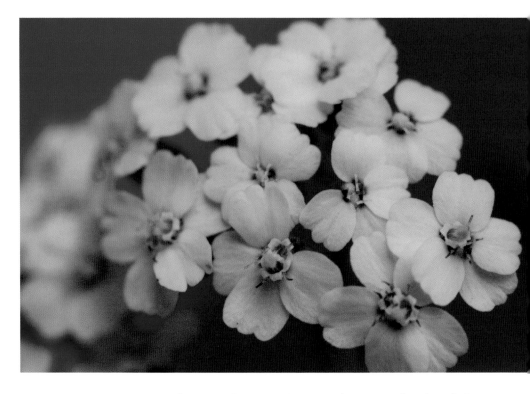

*... Any treatment for external and internal haemorrhage calls for the inclusion of Yarrow.... I cannot imagine dealing effectively with painful periods or with high blood pressure if the prescription did not include a small but positive amount of Yarrow.*
– Barker (2001)

But there is another range of bodily ills for which yarrow is well recommended, and this is in reducing fevers. By relaxing the skin, yarrow will open the pores to allow copious sweating and the release of toxins. Yarrow taken as tea or as a bath at the beginning of a fever or flu is an excellent way to reduce the body temperature. It is an herb for measles and chicken pox, and it is safe for children. It was once called "Englishman's quinine" for a claimed benefit for treating ague (a form of malaria).

The sweating / purifying / relaxing effects are enhanced, herbalists have found, by combining equal quantities of yarrow, peppermint, and elderflower in a tea, drunk as hot and as often as the patient can stand. The same mix works well as a skin lotion or in a bath. The equivalent mixture for high blood pressure is yarrow plus nettle and lime blossom, again taken as a tea.

Yarrow has various other health benefits, as befits its all-rounder status. Its effect on bodily fluids helps in cases of diarrhea and dysentery. It is effective for colic and blockages of the urogenital area, as also for stomach cramps, cystitis, arthritis, and rheumatism.

A yarrow lotion makes a good eyebath and stimulates the scalp, with traditional benefit to the hair; plugs of crushed leaves help to relieve toothache or earache.

Yarrow has a further dimension to its long human history: it is an herb of divination, used by the Druids for predicting the weather, by the Chinese for auguries (in the *Book of Changes* or *I Ching*), and by love-lorn English maidens for indicating who their true love would be. One chant from East Anglia links the yarrow of blood and the yarrow of foretelling:

*Yarroway, yarroway, bear a white blow/ If my love love me, my nose will bleed now.*

These were benign uses, but the past is not one-sided and yarrow also had a shadow side, being called the "devil's nettle" and "bad man's plaything." For the most part it was involved in sympathetic magic, as in its part in St John's day celebrations (see page 161).

All this virtue, and a little vice, comes with a tally of yarrow's profit and loss account. No question, it is one of the great presences in western herbalism. At the same time, some cautions should be noted.

Yarrow has a stimulating effect on uterine contractions, so is best avoided in pregnancy; prolonged use externally can, in some people, cause allergic rashes and make the skin ultra-sensitive to sunlight; large doses can cause headaches.

You should also be aware that the active constituents of yarrow vary from plant to plant and by locality. If you try yarrow for any of the uses we have outlined and it seems to be ineffective, go to another plant and use that.

*Milfoil is always the greatest boon, wherever it grows wild in the country.... It should on no account be weeded out. Like sympathetic people in human society, who have a favourable influence by their mere presence ... so milfoil, in a district where it is plentiful, works beneficially by its mere presence.*
*– Steiner (early 20th century)*

Yarrow by Maria Merian (1717)

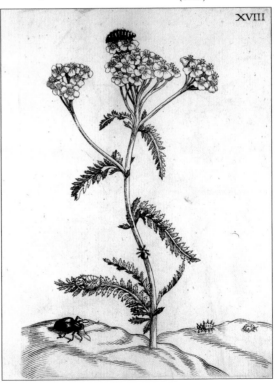

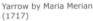

**Yarrow tea**
- colds and fevers
- scanty menstruation
- heavy periods
- menstrual clotting
- high blood pressure
- to tone varicose veins
- to prevent blood clots
- tension
- weak digestion

**Yarrow tincture**
- scanty menstruation
- heavy periods
- menstrual clotting
- high blood pressure
- to tone varicose veins
- to prevent blood clots
- tension
- weak digestion

**Fresh leaf**
- nosebleeds
- cuts and wounds

## Harvesting yarrow

Yarrow leaves are evergreen so can be harvested fresh almost whenever they are needed. To make a tincture or when drying for tea, it is best gathered while flowering. Yarrow accumulates particulates from vehicle exhausts because of the large surface area of its flowerhead and leaves, so it is best to pick it away from busy roads.

To dry your yarrow, hang whole stems in bunches or place them on brown paper in a warm dry place. Allow a month, and once they are dry, strip the leaves and flowers off the stems and crumble for use as a tea. Smaller stems can be chopped up with scissors, but the larger stems are usually discarded. Keep the leaves dry and you can use them for months, or find fresh leaves for a green tea.

### Yarrow tea

Use 1 heaped teaspoonful of **dried yarrow** per cup or mug of **boiling water**, and let it infuse for 10 minutes. Strain and drink hot.

**Dose:** For colds and feverish conditions, drink a cupful hot every two hours until there is an improvement, and continue drinking three cups a day until you are well. For chronic conditions, drink three cups a day. For fevers, yarrow combines well with mint and elderflower. Use externally as a wash for cuts, and as a hair rinse for a healthy scalp and shiny hair.

### Yarrow tincture

Chop up **fresh yarrow leaves and flowers**, and put in a jar. Pour in enough **vodka** to cover, put the lid on, and place the jar in a dark cupboard for two weeks. Shake it every few days. Strain and bottle.

**Dose:** 20 drops in water, three times a day.

### Ointment for hemorrhoids

Gently heat 1 oz **dried yarrow** and 1 oz **dried raspberry leaf** or 1 oz **horse chestnut leaf** with 1 cup **extra virgin olive oil** in a small saucepan for 15 minutes, stirring frequently. Strain out the herbs and return the oil to the pan. Add about 1 oz **beeswax** and stir until melted. Use enough beeswax to set the ointment – test a few drops on a cold saucer as you do when making jelly. If you live in a hot climate or it is summer, you will want to use more beeswax than if the weather is cold. If your ointment is too runny, you can melt it again and add more beeswax.

Apply the ointment externally a couple of times a day as needed. It can also be used on bruises, varicose veins, and thread veins.

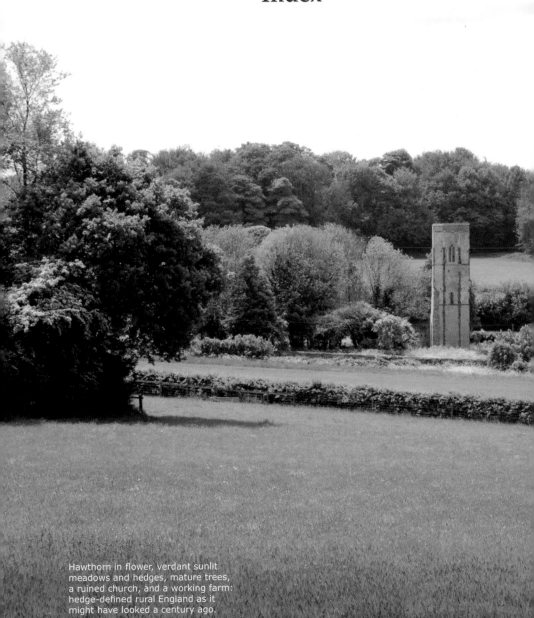

# Notes to the text
# Recommended reading
# Resources
# Index

Hawthorn in flower, verdant sunlit
meadows and hedges, mature trees,
a ruined church, and a working farm:
hedge-defined rural England as it
might have looked a century ago.

# Notes to the text

*Full citation given in first reference only, thereafter author and page number. Orginal year of publication is in square brackets; place of publication London unless otherwise noted*

**Preface [viii]:** Boerhaave's hat: Chris Howkins, *The Elder: The Mother Tree of Folklore* (Addlestone, Surrey, 1996), 28.

**Introduction [ix]:** Hew DV Prendergast & Helen Sanderson, *Britain's Wild Harvest: The Commercial Uses of Wild Plants and Fungi* (2004), 64.

**Harvesting from the wild [x]:** James Green, *The Herbal Medicine-Maker's Handbook: A Home Manual* (Berkeley, CA, 2000), 10; Steven Foster & James Duke, *A Field Guide to Medicinal Plants and Herbs: Of Eastern and Central North America* (Boston, MA, 1999); nettle and elderflower from William Woodville, *Medical Botany*, 4 vols (1790–3), courtesy of John Innes Foundation Historical Collections, Norwich.

Relevant North American legislation on harvesting wild plants is found in the US Plant Protection Act (PPA) of June 2000, which consolidates previous law. The US Department of Agriculture (USDA) is the federal agency responsible, through the PPA, for regulating the growing, sale, and import of commercial plants and for keeping a noxious weeds register. The USDA website, www.usda.gov, gives the links to state legislation.

The Endangered Species Listing Program of 1999 controls the federal schedule of endangered species. No such plant is included in this book.

There is no general law against harvesting wild plants unless they are endangered, threatened, or illegal. Ownership dictates whether you can legally harvest in a particular place, and usually the permission of the owner is required or advised. Picking in declared wilderness, state, and national parks and many freeways is usually forbidden. For an overview on protocols and common sense on harvesting, see the UK code of conduct on www.bsbi.org.uk.

**AGRIMONY [2–5]:** Woodville, *Medical Botany*, IV, 254, courtesy of John Innes Foundation Historical Collections, Norwich; Matthew Wood, *The Book of Herbal Wisdom* (Berkeley, CA, 1997), 85–92 passim; Anne Pratt, *The Flowering Plants and Ferns of Great Britain*, 5 vols (1857), II, 218; John Parkinson, *Theatrum Botanicum* (1640), 597.

**BILBERRY [6–11]:** "hunter-gatherer": Richard Mabey, *Food for Free* (2000 [1972]), 100–1; "mucky-mouth pies": Mabey, *Flora Britannica* (1997), 163; James Duke, *The Green Pharmacy* (Emmaus, PA, 1997), 318; Nicholas Culpeper, *Complete Herbal* (1995 [1653]), 33; Abbé Kneipp, quoted in Jean Palaiseul, *Grandmother's Secrets*, trans. Pamela Swinglehurst (1976 [1972]), 48; Mrs M Grieve, *A Modern Herbal*, ed. Mrs CF Leyel (1998 [1931]), 99–100; Geoffrey Grigson, *The Englishman's Flora* (1975 [1958]), 282.

**BIRCH [12–15]:** Baron Percy, quoted in Palaiseul, 50–1.

**BLACKBERRY, BRAMBLE [16–19]:** Walt Whitman, "Song of Myself" 2, stanza 31, *Leaves of Grass* (New York, 1855); Jonathan Roberts, *Cabbages & Kings* (2001), 17; Dennis Furnell, *Health from the Hedgerow* (1985), 44–5; Carol Belanger Grafton, *Medieval Herb, Plant and Flower Illustrations* [CD-Rom and book] (New York, 2004), image 165; Julian Barker, *The Medicinal Flora of Britain and Northwestern Europe* (West Wickham, Kent, 2001), 171.

**BURDOCK [20–23]:** "official": British Herbal Medical Association, *British Herbal Pharmacopoeia* (1996), 49; Green, *Herbal Medicine-Maker's Handbook*, 35.

**CHERRY [24–25]:** "Wildman" Steve Brill & Evelyn Dean, *Identifying and Harvesting Edible and Medicinal Plants* (New York, 2002 [1994]), 119; Grigson, 177.

**CHICKWEED [26–29]:** Brill & Dean, 138; Susun Weed, *Wise Woman Herbal: Healing Wise* (Woodstock, NY, 1989), 122.

**CLEAVERS [30–33]:** Culpeper, 73; Parkinson, 568; Maria Treben, *Health through God's Pharmacy* (Steyr, Austria, 1983 [1980]), 10–11; John Pughe, ed. & trans., *The Physicians of Myddfai* (Felinfach, Wales, 1993 [1861]), 444; John Evelyn, *Acetaria: A Discourse on Sallets* (1699 [Brooklyn, 1937]), 12.

**COLTSFOOT [34–37]:** Barker, 472; tobacco: Robert John Thornton, *A New Family Herbal* (1810), 711.

**COMFREY [38–41]:** names: Deni Bown, *The RHS Encyclopedia of Herbs & Their Uses* (1995), 206; Bocking 14: Henry Doubleday Research Association, www.gardenorganic.org.uk; Norfolk recipe: Book of Culinary Recipes, 1739–79 (Norfolk Record Office, RMN 4/5), fo. 4; Dr John R Christopher, *School of Natural Healing* (Springville, UT, 1996 [1976]), 337; Norman Grainger Bisset & Max Wichtl, eds, *Herbal Drugs and Phytopharmaceuticals*, 2nd edn (Stuttgart/Boca Raton, 2001 [1989]), 485; Weed, www.susunweed.com.

**COUCH GRASS [42–45]:** Culpeper, 93; "civice": Audrey Wynne Hatfield, *How to Enjoy Your Weeds* (Worcestershire, 1999 [1969]), 47; *King's American Dispensatory*, by Harvey Wickes Felter & John Uri Lloyd (1898), www.henriettesherbal.com; Parkinson, 1175; Bisset & Wichtl, 242.

**CURLED DOCK, YELLOW DOCK [46–49]:** Weeds Act 1959, www.defra.gov.uk; seeds: Maida Silverman, *A City Herbal*, 3rd edn (Woodstock, NY, 1997 [1977]), 57; chants: Roy Vickery, comp., *A Dictionary of Plant-Lore* (1995), 107; Tswana women: Margaret Roberts, *Margaret Roberts' Book of Herbs* (Johannesburg, 1983), 61; David E

Allen & Gabrielle Hatfield, *Medicinal Plants in Folk Tradition* (Portland, OR/ Cambridge, 2004), 98; Maria Sibylla Merian, *Erucarum ortus alimentum et paradoxa metamorphosis* (Amsterdam, c1717), courtesy of John Innes Foundation Historical Collections, Norwich; Culpeper, 91; old herbalists: Thomas Bartram, *Bartram's Encyclopedia of Herbal Medicine* (1998 [1995]), 459; "superlative remedy": Matthew Wood, *The Practice of Traditional Western Herbalism* (Berkeley, CA, 2004), 152; jaundice recipe: Mary Norwalk, *East Anglian Recipes*, 2nd edn (Dereham, 1996 [1976]), 40.

**DANDELION [50–55]:** English/ Chinese names: Silverman, 50–1, 53; William Coles, quoted in Silverman, 51; US salad industry: Brigitte Mars, *Dandelion Medicine* (Pownal, VT, 1999), 18; quotation, Mars, 1.

**ELDER [56–61]:** Chambers: quoted in Howkins, *The Elder*, 20; John Evelyn, *Sylva* (1664), ch. XX, 17, www. gutenberg.org; Ria Loohuizen, *The Elder in History, Myth and Cookery* (Totnes, 2005); cordials: Prendergast & Sanderson, 24–7; Norfolk recipe: Book of Culinary Recipes, 1739–79 (NRO, RMN 4/5), fo. 14.

**GUELDER ROSE, CRAMPBARK [62–63]:** Gerard: Grigson, 380; Rosemary Gladstar, *Herbal Healing for Women* (New York, 1993), 175, 239; Dr Christopher, 431.

**HAWTHORN [64–69]:** Pratt, II, 269; Dr Green: Bertram, 215; Jennings: HP Whitford et al., *A Treatise on Crataegus* (Cincinnati, 1917), www. herbaltherapeutics.net; Peter Conway, *Tree Medicine* (2001), 170; "Fair Maid": Blanche Fisher Wright, illus., *The Real Mother Goose* (New York, 1916), www. gutenberg.org; hawthorn berry leather: inspired by Ray Mears, "Wild Food," BBC2, 31.1.07.

**HONEYSUCKLE, WOODBINE [70–71]:** English woodland: Furnell, 98; twizzly canes: Katherine Kear, *Flower Wisdom* (2000), 89; yellow-flowered varieties: Christopher Hobbs (herbal

workshop); *shuan huang lian*: Duke, 93–4; Anne McIntyre, *The Complete Floral Healer* (1996), 147; Parkinson, 1461.

**HOPS [72–73]:** John Gerard, *The Herball*, ed. Marcus Woodward (1994 [1597]), 213; Laurel Dewey, *The Humorous Herbalist* (East Canaan, CT, 1996), 92; Evelyn, *Acetaria*, 19; George III: Mabey, *Flora Britannica*, 64; "official": *Br. Herbal Pharm.*, 106.

**HORSE CHESTNUT [74–77]:** "park": figure cited in *Independent*, 24.8.06; Turkey: McIntyre, 52; Chris Howkins, *Horse Chestnut* (Addlestone, 2005), 20–1; First World War: Howkins, 29–32; David Hoffmann, *Medical Herbalism* (Rochester, VT, 2003), 524.

**HORSERADISH [78–79]:** Parkinson, 861; Philippa Back, *The Illustrated Herbal* (1987), 75; John Pechey, *The Compleat Herbal of Physical Plants*, 2nd edn (1707 [1694]), 197.

**HORSETAIL [80–83]:** Furnell, 102–4; "drumsticks": Palaiseul, 154; "moth-eaten asparagus": Hatfield, *Weeds*, 75; Galen, quoted in Mrs Grieve, 421; Treben, 26–9.

**LIME, LINDEN [84–86]:** Barker, 237; Conway, 271.

**LYCIUM [87–91]:** David Winston & Steven Maimes, *Adaptogens* (Rochester, VT, 2007), 178–81; Lu Ji and Chinese saying, Winston & Maimes, 179; protecting UK hedgerows: Department for Environment, Food and Rural Affairs, www.defra.gov.uk 15.1.03; goji as food: Food Standards Authority, www.food.gov.uk 18.6.07; Duke of Argyll: Mabey, *Flora Britannica*, 300; aphrodisiac: Duke, 192.

**MALLOW [92–95]:** *Br. Herb. Pharm.*, 127–30 (leaf & root); Treben, 31–2; Cobbett, quoted in A. Lawson, *The Modern Farrier* [1842], 282–4; Gabrielle Hatfield, *Memory, Wisdom and Healing* (Stroud, 1999), 40–2; *Hortus Floridus* (1614–16), courtesy of John Innes Foundation Historical Collections, Norwich; Culpeper, 156, 159; mallow

tea: Richo Cech, *Making Plant Medicine* (Williams, OR, 2000), 182; "far from roads": Furnell, 122; Cicero: Clinton C. Gilroy, *The History of Silk, Cotton, Linen, Wool, and Other Fibrous Substances* (New York, 1843), 191–202, www. books.google.com.

**MEADOWSWEET [96–99]:** Turner: Grigson, 154; Chaucer: Mrs Grieve, 524; Parkinson, 593; Cuchulainn: Tess Darwin, *The Scots Herbal* (Edinburgh, 1996), 149; Palaiseul, 208; Cech, 183.

**MINT [100–03]:** "fishes": Palaiseul, 211; Gerard, 155; William Thomas Fernie, *Herbal Simples Approved for Modern Uses of Cure* (Philadelphia, 1897), 342, www.gutenberg. org; Parkinson, 35; "official": *Br. Herb. Pharm.*, 149; sekanjabin: adapted from traditional Persian recipes; Rumi: quoted in www.superluminal.com.

**MUGWORT [104–09]:** "female remedy": McIntyre, 57; northern saying: Susan Lavender & Anna Franklin, *Herb Craft* (Chieveley, 1996), 371; Sir John Hill, *The British Herbal* (1756), quoted in Keith Vincent Smith, *The Illustrated Earth Garden Herbal* (1979), 100; insecticide: Pughe, *Myddfai*, 53; Silverman: quote and *Leech-Book*, 92, 94; moxa: Thornton, 695; tobacco, Manx festival: Mabey, *Flora Britannica*, 370.

**MULLEIN [110–13]:** Odysseus: Homer, *The Odyssey*, trans. EV Rieu (Harmondsworth, 1979 [1946]), 163; quaker girls: Wood, *Herbal Wisdom*, 493; Hildegard: Wighard Strehlow & Gottfried Hertzka, *Hildegard of Bingen's Medicine*, trans. Karin Anderson Strehlow (Santa Fe, NM, 1988), 21; Dr Quinlan: Allen & Hatfield, 250; Michael Moore, *Medicinal Plants of the Mountain West* (Santa Fe, NM, 1979), 113; Dr Christopher, 345.

**NETTLE [114–19]:** "springtime herbalism": James Green, *The Male Herbal* (Freedom, CA, 1991), 92; Milarepa: *The Oxford Companion to Food*, ed. Alan Davidson (Oxford, 1999), 532; Dr HCA Vogel, *The Nature Doctor* (Edinburgh, 1990 [1952]), 369;

Hatfield, *Weeds*, 93; Merian, *Erucarum ortus*; nettle-eating: Piers Warren, *101 Uses for Stinging Nettles* (2006), 71; Sir John Harington, *Regimen Sanitatis Salernitanum* (1607), quoted in Keith GR Wheeler, *A Natural History of Nettles* (Victoria, BC, 2005), 48; Weed, 171; Duke, 371.

**OAK [120–23]:** "necessary": Grigson, 269; bark "official": *Br. Herb. Pharm.*, 145; Moore, 116; "half-pay": Grigson, 273; Hoffmann, *Medical*, 497; German: Bisset & Wichtl, 403; Culpeper, 182.

**PELLITORY OF THE WALL [124–25]:** Parkinson, 437; Culpeper, 192; Norfolk recipe: Anon., *Archdale Palmer's Recipes 1659–1672* (Wymondham, Leics, n.d.), unpaginated; asthma weed: www.weeds.org.au; Mrs Grieve, 624.

**PLANTAIN [126–31]:** sacred herb: Grigson, 356; lawns: Ken Fern, *Plants for a Future*, 2nd edn (East Meon, Hants, 2000 [1997]), 144; footprint: Lesley Gordon, *A Country Herbal* (Exeter, 1980), 135–6; *Archdale Palmer's Recipes*; "Indian bandaid": JT & Michael Garrett, *Medicine of the Cherokee* (Rochester, VT, 1996), 57; Abbé Kneipp, quoted in Palaiseul, 250; Bessie Smith: Darwin, 138; Dr Christopher, 57; Merian, *Erucarum ortus*.

**RAMSONS, BEAR GARLIC [132–35]:** Hippocrates: www.bmj.com; Mrs Grieve, 344; Abbé Kuenzle, quoted in Treben, 37; Plants for a Future database: www.pfaf.org.

**RASPBERRY [136–38]:** Ida: *Oxford Companion to Food*, 653; Juliette de Baïracli Levy, *The Complete Herbal Book for the Dog* (1971 [1955]), 59; John Parkinson, *Paradisi in Sole: Paradisus Terrestris* (1629 [New York, 1976]), 558.

**RED CLOVER [139–41]:** Scott: *Guy Mannering* (1815), ch. 3; Hatfield, *Weeds*, 38–9; Dr Christopher, 61; Matthew Wood, pers. comm., 9 Jan 2008; "official": *Br. Herb. Pharm.*, 161; phyto-estrogens: Ruth Trickey, *Women, Hormones & the Menstrual Cycle*, 2nd edn (Crows Nest, NSW, 2003 [1998]), 402–4.

**RED POPPY [142–45]:** and war: eg Grigson, 57; Myddfai: Pughe, 414; Pechey, 192.

**ROSEBAY WILLOWHERB, FIREWEED [146–49]:** Singerweed: Roy Vickery, *Plant Lore Notes and News* (Dec. 1998); Roger Phillips, *Wild Food* (1983), 77; Felter & Lloyd, *King's American Dispensatory*, www.henriettesherbal.com; Carol Rudd, *Flower Essences* (Shaftesbury, Dorset, 1998), 52.

**SELF-HEAL [150–54]:** Chinese background: Henry C Lu, *Chinese Natural Cures* (New York, 1994), 204–5; Parkinson, 528; *Brunella*: Malcolm Stuart (ed.), *The Encyclopedia of Herbs and Herbalism* (New York, 1979), 247; Gerard, 145; Duke, 256–7, 273.

**SHEPHERD'S PURSE [155–57]:** Barker, 146; Ryokan poem: trans. John Stevens, *Dewdrops on a Lotus Leaf: Zen Poems of Ryokan* (Boston, MA, 1996).

**ST JOHN'S WORT [158–63]:** "hyperikon": Wood, *Book*, 307; Parkinson, 574; Mrs Grieve, 708; MAO: Dewey, 137; use in Germany: Larry Katzenstein, *Secrets of St John's Wort* (1998); Alfred Lear Huxford: quoted in Anne Pratt, *Wild Flowers* (1852), 109; herbs of St John: Grigson, 85–6; Klamath weed: Grigson, 88–9; Australasia: Sir Edward Salisbury, *Weeds & Aliens* (1961), 208.

**SWEET CICELY [164–66]:** Gerard, 244; Culpeper, 66; Furnell, 165.

**TEASEL [167–69]:** bath of Venus, eg, Allen & Hatfield, 275; fulling: Mrs Grieve, 754; TCM: Dan Bensky & Andrew Gamble, *Chinese Herbal Medicine Materia Medica*, rev. edn (Seattle, WA, 1993 [1986]), 349; Wood, *Book*, 234–7; lyme: Stephen Harrod Buhner, *Healing Lyme* (Randolph, VT, 2005).

**VERVAIN [170–72]:** prayer: TF Thiselton Dyer, *The Folklore of Plants* (Llanerch, Wales, 1994 [1889]), 285; Mydffai: Pughe, 448–9; Parkinson, 676; marriage and *verbenarius*, McIntyre, 233; Pechey, 241; Pratt, IV, 210.

**WHITE DEADNETTLE, ARCHANGEL [173–75]:** names: Mrs Grieve, 580; Gerard, 158; "too common" and quote: Barker, 370.

**WILD LETTUCE [176–77]:** wild vs commercial: Brill & Dean, 246; lactucarium and 1771: Stuart, 210; "official": *Br. Herb. Pharm.*, 185; Galen and "eunuch's plant": Palaiseul, 184; Min: Penelope Ody, *Essential Guide to Natural Home Remedies* (2002), 128; "o'er much lettuce": www.easyhomeremedy.com.

**WILD ROSE [178–83]:** Vitamin C and wartime use: Mabey, 192; Anacreon: quoted in Maggie Tisserand, *Essential Oils for Lovers* (1999 [1993]), 97; Bartholomew: quoted in Eleanour Sinclair Rohde, *The Old English Herbals* (New York, 1971 [1922]), 49; Pechey, 202; Milto: Tisserand, 96; Pliny: Stuart, 253; dagger and other names: Back, 55; love-charm, Germany: Pamela Allardice, *Aphrodisiacs & Love Magic* (Bridport, Dorset, 1989), 21; gall: Grigson, 174; Askham's Herbal: Rohde, 60.

**WILLOW [184–85]:** Culpeper, 272; Ben-Erik van Wyk *et al.*, *Medicinal Plants of South Africa* (Pretoria, 1997), 222 [re *Salix mucronata*, wild willow]; www.aspirin-foundation.com, www.pfaf.org.

**WILLOWHERB [186–87]:** Treben, 49; Gerard, 114; Parkinson, 549.

**WOOD BETONY [188–91]:** Culpeper, 30, 31–2; Pratt, IV, 189; Parkinson, 616; *Grete Herball*: Rohde, 72; John Clare: quoted in Pratt, *Wild Flowers*, www.books.google.com.

**YARROW [192–96]:** "herb for women": Treben, 50; "cure-all": Barker, 460; Margaret Roberts, 31; Hoffmann, *Medical*, 523; Barker, 460; East Anglian saying: quoted in Keith Vincent Smith, 136; Rudolf Steiner [n.d.]: quoted in Smith, 136; Merian, *Erucarum ortus*.

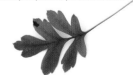

# Recommended reading

Back, Philippa. *The Illustrated Herbal*. London, 1987

Barker, Julian. *The Medicinal Flora of Britain & Northwestern Europe: A Field Guide*. West Wickham, Kent, 2001

Bartram, Thomas. *Bartram's Encyclopedia of Herbal Medicine*. London, 1998 [1995]

Blamey, Marjorie, Richard & Alastair Fitter. *Wild Flowers of Britain & Ireland*. London, 2003

Brill, "Wildman" Steve, with Evelyn Dean. *Identifying and Harvesting Edible and Medicinal Plants in Wild (and Not so Wild) Places*. New York, 1994

Buhner, Stephen Harrod. *Sacred Plant Medicine: The Wisdom in Native American Herbalism*. Rochester, VT, 2006 [1996]

Cech, Richo. *Making Plant Medicine*. Williams, OR, 2000

Chevallier, Andrew. *The Encyclopedia of Medicinal Plants*. London, 1996
—— *Herbal Remedies*. London, 2007

Duke, James A. *The Green Pharmacy*. Emmaus, PA, 1997

Foster, Steven & James Duke. *A Field Guide to Medicinal Plants & Herbs: Of Eastern & Central North America*. Boston, MA, 1999

Green, James. *The Herbal Medicine-Maker's Handbook: A Home Manual*. Berkeley, CA, 2002

Grieve, Mrs M, ed. and introd. Mrs CF Leyel. *A Modern Herbal: The Medicinal, Culinary, Cosmetic and Economic Properties, Cultivation and Folklore of Herbs, Grasses, Fungi, Shrubs and Trees with all their Modern Scientific Uses*. London, 1998 [1931]; online at www.botanical.com

Grigson, Geoffrey. *The Englishman's Flora*. London, 1975 [1958]

Hatfield, Audrey Wynne. *How to Enjoy Your Weeds*. Worcestershire, 1999 [1969]

Hoffmann, David. *The New Holistic Herbal: A Herbal Celebrating the Wholeness of Life*, 2nd edn. Shaftesbury, Dorset, 1986 [1983]

Mabey, Richard. *Flora Britannica*. London, 1996
—— *Food for Free*. London, 2001 [1972]

McIntyre, Anne. *The Complete Floral Healer: The Healing Power of Flowers through Herbalism, Aromatherapy, Homeopathy and Flower Essences*. London, 1996

Moore, Michael. *Medicinal Plants of the Mountain West*. Santa Fe, NM, 1979

—— *Medicinal Plants of the Desert and Canyon West*. Santa Fe, NM, 1989

Palaiseul, Jean. *Grandmother's Secrets: Her Green Guide to Health from Plants*. Trans. Pamela Swinglehurst. London, 1973 [1972]

Phillips, Roger. *Wild Food*. London, 1983

Silverman, Maida. *A City Herbal: Lore, Legend, & Uses of Common Weeds*, 3rd edn. Woodstock, NY, 1997 [1977]

Treben, Maria. *Health through God's Pharmacy: Advice and Experiences with Medicinal Herbs*. Steyr, Austria, 1983 [1982]

Uphoff, Karin C. *Botanical Body Care: Herbs and Natural Healing for Your Whole Body*. Fort Bragg, CA, 1997

Wood, Matthew. *The Book of Herbal Wisdom*. Berkeley, CA, 1997
—— *The Practice of Traditional Western Herbalism: Basic Doctrine, Energetics and Classification*. Berkeley, CA, 2004
—— *The Earthwise Herbal: A Complete Guide to Old World Medicinal Plants*. Berkeley, CA, 2008

# Resources

## Supplies

You can find most of what you need in health stores, grocery, and hardware stores.

Frontier Natural Products Co-op
PO Box 299
3021 78th St
Norway, IA 52318
Phone: (800) 669-3275
www.frontiercoop.com
Beeswax, empty capsules, etc.;
also herbs, spices, and body care

Neals Yard Remedies
www.nyrusa.com
www.nealsyardremedies.com
Beeswax, lanolin, brown glass
bottles; also herbs and body care

## Seeds and plants

Horizon Herbs
PO Box 69
Williams, OR 97544
Phone: (541) 846-6704
www.horizonherbs.com
Run by herbalist Richo Cech, author of *Making Plant Medicine*; excellent selection of medicinal plants and seeds; comprehensive annual catalog

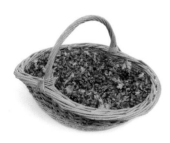

## Plant information

American Botanical Council
http://abc.herbalgram.org
Provides information on medicinal plants; publishes *Herbalgram*

American Herb Association
www.ahaherb.com

Hedgerow Medicine
www.hedgerowmedicine.com
Updates to this book, recipes etc.

Henriette Kress
www.henriettesherbal.com
Herbal information website

Plantlife International
www.plantlife.org.uk
Wild-plant conservation charity

Plants for a Future
www.pfaf.org
Information on edible, medicinal, and other useful plants

The Herb Society of America
www.herbsociety.org
Promotes the knowledge, use, and delight of herbs; publishes The *Herbarist* magazine

United Plantsavers
PO Box 400, East Barre, VT 05649
Tel. (802) 476-6467
http://unitedplantsavers.org/
Charity protecting native medicinal plants of North America

USDA Plants Database
http://plants.usda.gov
Distribution maps for wild plants in the US and Canada (including all those in this book)

## Herbal medicine-making

For more detailed information on making your own herbal medicines, we recommend these two books.

*Making Plant Medicine* by Richo Cech. Williams, OR, 2000

*The Herbal Medicine-Maker's Handbook: A Home Manual* by James Green. Berkeley, CA, 2002

## Finding an herbal practitioner

Word of mouth is often the best way to find a good herbalist. Ask friends or your local health food stores to see who they can recommend.

You can also contact the professional associations below for a listing of practicing members.

American Herbalists Guild (AHG)
141 Nob Hill Road,
Cheshire, CT 06410
Phone: (203) 272-6731
www.americanherbalistsguild.com

Canadian Herbalist Association of BC (CHAofBC)
www.chaofbc.ca

The Ontario Herbalists Association
www.herbalists.on.ca

# Index

**Bold** *type indicates a main entry*

A
abscess 52, 95, 151
*Achillea millefolium* **192–6**
acidity 98, 99, 180; *see also* stomach acid
acne xviii, 20, 23, 48, 52, 53, 140, 141, 180
acne rosacea 76, 130
addiction 3, 122, 189
adenoids 31
ADHD (attention deficit hyperactivity disorder) 68
adrenals 117
*Aesculus hippocastanum* **74–7**
age spots 53
aging 7, 52, 53, 90, 164, 172, 190, 191
*Agrimonia eupatoria* **2–5**
agrimony **2–5**; harvesting 5; recipes 5
ague 185, 194
AIDS 88, 152, 161
alcoholism 122
ale 72, 106, 125, 144
alkaloids 36, 39, 40, 82
all-heal **150–4**
allergies 115, 117, 125, 128, 130, 152, 163, 195
*Allium ursinum* **132–5**
ambrosia 15
anal fissure 122
anaphrodisiac 102, 177, 185
anemia 18, 25, 33, 48, 49, 115–16, 117, 137, 138
angina 66, 69
Anglo-Saxons 8, 42, 47, 48, 107, 115, 122, 127, 139, 167, 179, 181
aniseed 164
ankle: sprained 5; swollen 53
anorexia 23, 73
anthocyanins 7, 25
antibacterial 8, 119, 134, 152, 193
antibiotic xv, 148
anti-fungal 102, 108, 115, 134
antihistamine 115, 128
anti-inflammatory 38, 39, 98, 123
anti-microbial 44, 71, 79, 122, 193
antioxidant 7, 11, 25, 88, 137, 152
antiseptic xv, 9, 71, 79, 102, 122, 123, 162
anti-tussive 24
antiviral 102, 151, 152, 161, 180
anxiety 69, 84, 85, 86, 109, 144, 145, 172, 189, 191
apéritif 166
aphrodisiac 90, 91, 115, 118, 171, 181
appendicitis 4
appetite 23, 73, 102, 103, 109, 164, 166, 190, 191
Archangel **173–5**
*Arctium* spp. **20–3**
*Armoracia rusticana* **78–9**
*Artemisia vulgaris* **104–9**
arteries, hardening 53, 66, 69, 84
arteriosclerosis 53, 66, 69, 84
arthritis 14, 15, 22, 23, 25, 38, 41, 54, 55, 79, 116, 138, 162, 169, 174, 185, 195

aspirin 70, 97–8, 184–5
asthma 4, 28, 37, 71, 115, 125
astringency 4, 5, 8, 18, 88, 98, 122, 137, 145, 147–8, 174, 180, 185, 187
atherosclerosis 88
athlete's foot 4, 5
athletic performance 68
Australia 17, 42, 125, 151
Ayurveda 48, 102, 104

B
Bach, Dr Edward 3, 77, 170
backache xviii, 5, 41, 63, 99, 112, 113, 162, 167, 185
bad breath 102
baths xviii, 5, 29, 59, 71, 83, 85, 94, 103, 122, 169, 194
bear garlic 68, **132–5**
bedwetting 4, 8, 53, 83, 158, 163
beer xv, 14, 55, 61, 76, 96, 106, 114
betony: *see* wood betony
*Betula pendula* **12–15**
bilberry **6–11**, 83, 156, 187; harvesting 6–7; recipes 11
bile 48, 52
birch **12–15**, 18; harvesting 15; recipes 15
bites 27, 48, 85, 95, 106, 122, 127, 128, 130, 174, 180
bitterness 4, 23, 52, 73, 76, 107, 122, 147, 176
blackberry 7, 11, **16–19**, 91, 141; harvesting 17; recipes 19
bladder: irritable 4, 9, 33, 44, 45, 82, 83, 125, 155, 156, 159, 187; stone 14, 182
bleeding 3, 4, 117, 122, 129, 130, 140, 148, 150, 151, 156, 157, 171, 174, 180, 185, 193
blisters 33, 53
bloating 102, 134, 161
blood 20, 37, 48, 52, 64, 82, 115, 132, 134, 140
blood poisoning 128, 129
blood pressure 53, 63, 66, 68, 69, 84, 86, 87, 115, 117, 140, 152, 156, 157, 194, 196
blood sugars 11, 115, 117
bog myrtle 72, 106
boils xviii, 18, 20, 23, 37, 48, 79, 85, 95, 112, 113, 130, 134, 171, 180, 181
bowels: inflammation 99; regulation 174; sluggish 49, 52, 95, 134, 148, 149
BPH (benign prostate hyperplasia) 174; *see also* prostate
bramble **16–19**, 91
breast: cancer 53, 141; cysts 33
brewing 72, 106
bronchitis 24, 25, 28, 37, 39, 44, 70, 71, 113, 129, 130, 140, 141
broth 27, 53, 111
bruises 23, 27, 39, 41, 59, 162, 174, 175, 191, 193, 196
buchu 83, 156
Buerger's disease 66
burdock **20–3**, 32, 33; recipes 23
burns 4, 5, 23, 27, 33, 85, 118, 122, 124, 130, 171, 174, 175
bursitis 41
butters xvii, 19

C
calcium 66, 90, 137
California poppy 73
calming 84, 108, 189, 190
cancer 7, 22, 32, 53, 88, 137, 140, 141
candida 148
capillaries 31, 77, 88, 91, 193
*Capsella bursa-pastoris* **155–7**; recipes 157
cardiac disease 115
cataract 8, 10, 88
catarrh 59, 79, 174, 175
cellulite 14, 15
*Chamerion angustifolium* **146–9**
chamomile 53, 111
cheese 29, 115, 119, 135
cherry, wild sweet 7, **24–5**, 61; recipes 25
chest 28, 59, 112, 113
chicken pox 194
chickweed **26–9**, 53, 128; recipes 29
chilblains 59, 83, 113, 122
childbirth 104, 138, 156, 190
children 76, 85, 98, 102, 128, 140, 141, 145, 148, 149, 172, 179, 194
chills 4, 191
China 30, 52, 87, 88, 90, 91, 104, 195
cholesterol 53, 66, 88, 91, 140
chronic fatigue syndrome (CFS) 169, 170, 185
chronic venous insufficiency (CVI) 76
circulation 59, 63, 64, 66, 68, 69, 77, 84, 88, 115, 132, 134, 167, 169, 191
claudication 66, 69
cleavers **30–3**; recipes 33
colds: *see* common cold
colic 85, 102, 116, 134, 166, 177
colitis 28, 48, 129, 134, 180, 189
coltsfoot xvii, **34–7**, 140; recipes 37
comfrey 27, 36, **38–41**; harvesting 40; recipes 41
Commission E 44, 122
common cold 18, 19, 25, 59, 60, 61, 71, 79, 85, 86, 94, 102, 103, 137, 138, 172, 179, 183, 185, 191, 196
compresses xviii, 172
concentration 190, 191
congestion 28, 59
conjunctivitis 4
connective tissue 82
constipation 4, 25, 48, 49, 54, 63, 95, 129, 130, 141, 174
contraceptive pill 159
convalescence 117, 166, 170, 180, 191
convulsions 28
cooling 151, 172, 179, 181
cordials 18, 58, 60, 61
corn marigold 161
corns 53
cornsilk 156
couch grass **42–5**, 83, 156, 187; recipes 45
cough 24, 25, 27, 36–7, 61, 79, 85, 94, 95, 102, 112, 113, 117, 118, 124, 129, 130, 141, 144, 145, 176, 177
crampbark **62–3**
cramps 63, 71, 85, 111, 138, 140, 174, 181, 195
*Crataegus* spp. **64–9**

creams 14, 153
Crohn's disease 73, 134
croup 71, 140
Culpeper, Nicholas 48, 124, 171, 188
curled dock 46–9, 141; harvesting 49; recipes 49
cuts 18, 38, 93, 95, 117, 122, 130, 134, 138, 148, 149, 150, 153, 174, 175, 192–3, 196
cystitis 4, 5, 14, 15, 32, 43, 45, 82, 83, 98, 124, 125, 174, 175, 195
cysts 33, 141

D
dandelion 14, 20, 22, 23, 32, 33, **50–5**; recipes 54–5
dandruff 22
decoctions xiii–xiv, xviii, 20, 23, 24, 82, 83, 111, 118, 119, 122, 124
depression 73, 108, 159–60, 162, 180, 189
detoxing 14, 15, 22, 48, 52
diabetes 9, 115, 152
diarrhea 3, 5, 8, 18, 19, 25, 48, 59, 70, 85, 97, 98, 117, 122, 129, 137, 138, 148, 149, 151, 159, 174, 175, 180, 185, 187, 195
digestion 4, 23, 33, 39, 52, 53, 54, 73, 79, 85, 101–3, 107, 108, 112, 117, 122, 145, 148, 164, 166, 171, 172, 189, 191, 196
digestive system 85, 129, 138, 180
digitalis 66
Dioscorides 27, 36, 189
*Dipsacus fullonum* **167–9**
diuretic 8, 22, 53, 59, 73, 82, 124, 179, 182
diverticulitis 99
divination 104, 195
dock 22, 32, 33, 128; common/broad-leaved 46, 47; curled: *see* curled dock
douches xviii, 122, 174, 175, 180
dreams 104, 108, 109
dropsy 14, 124–5
Duke of Argyll's tea plant **87–91**
dyeing 7, 8
dysentery 3, 8, 18, 48, 122, 180, 195

E
earache 31, 102, 112, 113
ecchymosis 155, 156
Eclectics 148, 149
escin 74, 76
eczema 14, 15, 20, 23, 27, 53, 54, 128, 141
edema 14, 76, 77, 124
elder xv, 7, 11, 24, 25, **56–61**, 63, 65, 102, 115, 128, 172, 180, 196, 196; dwarf 161; recipes 59–61
electuaries xvi, 99, 118, 124
*Elytrigia repens* **42–5**
embrocations xviii
emphysema 102
energy, low 22, 33
enteritis 48, 148
epilepsy 22, 170
*Epilobium* spp. **186–7**
*Equisetum arvense* **80–3**
essential oils xvii–xviii, 107, 180
estrogen 72, 140
eucalyptus 71
extremities, cold 88
eyesight 6, 8, 10, 11, 27, 52, 88, 91, 122, 134, 151, 191
eyewash 4, 5, 59, 158, 167, 180

F
fears 58, 162, 189
feet 103, 122, 129, 130
fennel 36, 37, 111, 123
fever 4, 15, 19, 58, 59, 60, 70, 71, 79, 84, 86, 97, 102, 115, 141, 148, 151, 152, 153, 172, 179, 184, 191, 193, 194, 196
fibromyalgia 14, 15, 169, 185
*Filipendula ulmaria* **96–9**
fireweed **146–9**
first aid 5, 27, 127–8, 130, 151, 174, 192–3
flashes: *see* hot flashes
flatulence 102, 103, 107, 109, 134, 164, 144, 174
flavonoids 7, 68
flower essences xvii, 3, 29, 77, 148, 154, 163, 169
flu (influenza) 19, 69, 61, 71, 79, 85, 86, 103, 137, 138, 151, 153, 179, 185, 194
fluid retention 15, 33, 54, 59, 77, 117, 124, 125
fomentations xviii
foxglove 39
fractures, bone 38, 39, 41, 82, 94, 112, 113
France 7, 53, 72, 93, 107, 161, 162, 193
freckles 53, 59
fructose 13

G
galangal 78
*Galium* 30
gall (tree) 120, 182
gallbladder 28, 44, 52, 53, 161, 190
gallstones 44, 52, 102
gangrene 128
gargle 138, 152, 153, 180
garlic 68; *see also* ramsons
gastritis 28, 189
gastroenteritis 8, 134
gastrointestinal problems 94, 174
Gerard, John 63, 107, 171
Germany 72, 122, 156, 160
ghees xvii, 99
ginger 68, 78
gingivitis 19
ginkgo 4
glands, swollen 31, 32, 33, 41, 112, 113, 141, 150, 151
glaucoma 8, 88
glycerine xv, xvi, 61, 71, 145, 182
glycerite xv, xvi, 10, 11, 25, 59, 60, 61, 99, 145, 180, 182
goitre 32, 151
goji berries **87–8**, 90–1
goose grass **30–3**
gout 14, 15, 23, 25, 44, 54, 64, 98, 116, 117, 185
gravel, urinary 15, 44, 125
Graves' disease 152
Greeks 28, 36, 105, 116, 133, 137, 177
griping 107, 109, 164, 166, 177
groin 48
ground ivy 72
guelder rose **62–3**, 185; harvesting 63; recipes 63
gums 4, 5, 18, 48, 98, 122, 123, 128, 138, 140, 162
gut: flora 88; infection 134; tension 190
gut instinct 159, 190

H
hair 53, 82, 83, 117, 196
hayfever 59, 66, 96, 115, 125, 128
hawthorn 7, 18, **64–9**, 156, 157, 182, 191; recipes 68–9
headaches xviii, 53, 63, 70, 86, 97, 102, 103, 172, 185, 189, 191, 195
heart 53, 64–9, 102, 134, 180
heartburn 98, 99, 161
heart disease 66
hedgerows ix, x
hemorrhage 194
hemorrhoids 9, 76, 113, 122, 130, 156, 191, 192, 196
hemostatic 117, 156
hepatic veno-occlusive disease 40
hepatitis 52
hernia, hiatus 99
herpes 14, 125, 151, 152
hiccups 102
Hildegard of Bingen 22, 111
HIV 22, 125, 161, 180
hives 102
hoarseness 111
homeopathic treatment 39, 77, 85, 122
honeys, herbal xv, xvi
honeysuckle **70–1**; recipes 71
hops xv, **72–3**, 106, 145, 177; recipes 73
hormone-balancing 171, 180
horse chestnut **74–7**, 196; recipes 77
horseradish 68, **78–9**, 191; harvesting 78; recipes 79
horsetail **80–3**, 156, 187; recipes 83
hot flashes 59, 71, 73, 86, 140, 141, 151, 153, 172
*Humulus lupulus* **72–3**
hyperactivity 73, 172
hypericin 158, 159
*Hypericum perforatum* **158–63**
hypoglycemia 9
hypothyroidism 152

I
immune system 22, 39, 88, 115, 151, 152, 179
impotence 87, 181
incontinence 4, 53, 82, 83
indigestion 79, 95, 98, 99, 102, 103, 164, 166
infection 59, 115, 119, 127, 130, 179
inflammation xviii, 7, 18, 27, 37, 59, 88, 119, 122, 128, 140, 152, 167, 169, 172, 179, 185, 190
influenza: *see* flu
infused oils xvii, xviii, 14, 15, 16, 41, 55, 153, 161, 162
infusions xiii–xiv, xviii, 5, 8–9, 11, 14, 15, 16, 19, 27, 29, 31–2, 36, 37, 39, 43, 45, 59, 85, 86, 94, 99, 103, 113, 115, 116, 117, 125, 130, 137, 138, 141, 149, 151, 153, 171–2, 174, 175, 191, 194, 196
insomnia 64, 72, 73, 85, 86, 144, 145, 162, 177, 180, 189, 191
insulin 7
Ireland 6, 97, 139–40
iron (mineral) 48, 90, 116, 137
irritable bowel syndrome (IBS) 63, 73, 95, 129, 130, 134, 145, 148, 175, 189
Isle of Man 6, 107, 108
itches 27, 28, 29, 112
ivy 16, 161

J
jams 7, 8, 18
Japan 20, 157
jaundice 44, 48, 49, 52, 159, 161
jet lag 162
joints, pain in xviii, 5, 38, 41, 55, 79, 92, 98, 99, 167, 169

K
kidney 20, 28, 52, 82, 83, 87, 116, 117, 118, 155, 167, 171; stone 4, 14, 15, 44, 45, 124, 181
knitbone **38–41**

L
lactation 47, 115, 117, 137, 185
*Lactuca virosa* **176–7**
lactucarium 176
*Lamium album* **173–5**
laryngitis 44, 113, 122
lavender 55
laxative 25, 48, 94, 95, 141
leaf oil 77
leather, fruit 68
leprosy 22
leucorrhea 122, 174, 175
ligaments 39, 41, 87
lime 68, **84–6**, 115, 145, 156, 157, 172, 194; recipes 86
linden **84–6**
liniments xviii, 63
lipoma 151
liver 4, 20, 28, 40, 44, 48, 49, 52, 53, 54, 87, 88, 107, 151, 161, 162, 167, 171, 190
*Lonicera periclymenum* **70–1**
loosestrife 187
lotion 77, 194
lungs 28, 53, 159
lupus 169
lycium 11, **87–91**; harvesting 90–1; recipes 91
Lyme disease 169
lymphatic system 31, 48, 52, 112, 113, 171; cancer 141

M
macular degeneration 10, 11, 88
malaria 87, 97, 108, 185, 194
mallow **92–5**; harvesting 94, 95; recipes 95
*Malva sylvestris* 53, **92–5**
manganese 137
MAO (monoamine oxidase) 160
marjoram 111
marshmallow 27, 95
massage 14, 15, 85, 117
mastitis 41
ME (myalgic encephalomyelitis) 169, 170, 185
mead 96
meadowsweet **96–9**, 184, 185; harvesting 99; recipes 99
measles 194
memory 134, 190, 191
menopause 52, 59, 60, 68, 71, 73, 84, 86, 140, 141, 153, 159, 162, 172, 182
menstruation 48, 52, 63, 73, 85, 104, 108, 109, 137, 138, 148, 150, 153, 156, 159, 172, 174, 175, 177, 181, 185, 190, 193, 194, 196
*Mentha aquatica* **100–3**
midges 106

migraine 63, 86, 102, 189, 193
minerals 26, 92, 115, 118
mint 59, **100–3**, 115, 128, 196; recipes 103
miscarriage 63, 102, 108
moths, clothes 106, 109
mouth ulcers 18, 19, 122, 123, 130, 138, 148, 149, 152, 153
mouthwash 128, 138, 149, 151, 153, 180
moxibustion 107
mucilage 39, 94, 129
mucous membrane 79, 122, 129
mucus 39, 94, 145, 155
mugwort **104–9**, 161; harvesting 109; recipes 109
mullein 36, **110–13**, 189; harvesting 113; recipes 113
mumps 112, 113
muscle tension/pain xviii, 4, 5, 14, 15, 39, 41, 55, 63, 79, 162, 169, 172, 177, 185, 191
mustard 78, 79
Mydffai, physicians of 106, 171
*Myrrhis odorata* **164–6**
myrtle 106

N
nails 82, 83
narcotic 73, 112, 143, 144
Native Americans 27, 106, 122, 127, 129, 147
nausea 102, 103, 138
neck, stiff 55, 151
nephritis 124
nervous disorders 63, 144, 145, 162, 169, 170; system 108, 112, 158, 171, 180; tension 86, 145, 172
nettle xv, 32, 33, 47, 59, 91, **114–19**, 173, 187, 194; harvesting 117, 119; recipes 117–19
nettle rash 33, 116
neuralgia 162
neuropathy 162
New Zealand 16–17, 20
nosebleeds 156, 192–3, 196

O
oak **120–3**; recipes 123
oatmeal 28, 29
oil, flower 112, 113
ointments xvii, 14, 33, 41, 59, 191, 196
opium 176; opium poppy 143, 144
osteoporosis 82, 138, 140
over-excitement 145, 177
overindulgence 54
oxalic acid 98
oxymels xvi, 19, 103, 138

P
pain relief 4, 97, 98, 112, 116, 118, 128, 144, 145, 153, 155, 161, 177, 185
palpitations 102
pancreas 52
*Parietaria judaica* **124–5**
Parkinson, John 3, 4, 107, 111, 124
passionflower 73
pasta 114
pellitory of the wall 83, **124–5**, 187; recipes 125
pelvic inflammation 85
pennyroyal 102
peppermint xvii, 100, 101–2, 194
pesto 26, 27, 114, 134

phlebitis 41
phyto-estrogens 140, 141
piles 28, 47, 113, 124
pillow 72, 73, 104, 106, 162, 191
pituitary gland 171
plague 66, 94, 95, 164
*Plantago lanceolata* xviii, **126–31**
*Plantago major* **126–31**, 161
*Plantago media* **126–31**
plantain 47, **126–31**; harvesting 130; recipes 130
plantar fasciitis 112, 129, 130
pleurisy 113
Pliny the Elder 36, 107, 181
PMT (premenstrual tension) 52, 172
polymyalgia rheumatica 185
porridge 114
potassium 14, 52, 53
poultices xviii, 20, 23, 27, 28, 33, 37, 39, 41, 79, 93, 95, 111, 112, 113, 135, 148, 149, 174, 175
powder 117, 123
pregnancy 102, 108, 137, 138, 155, 159, 195
premature ejaculation 73
prolapse 155, 156, 157, 190
prostate 23, 45, 82, 83, 116, 119, 124, 148; cancer 141, 156, 174, 186, 187
prostatitis 44
protection 16, 29, 64, 108, 111, 159, 161, 163, 164, 188, 189
Prozac 160
*Prunella vulgaris* **150–4**
*Prunus avium* 7, **24–5**
psoriasis 15, 20, 23, 33, 54, 141
psyllium 129
purgative 48, 95
pyrrolizidene alkaloids 36, 39, 40

Q
Quakers 111
*Quercus robur* **120–3**
quinine 74, 194
quinsy 151

R
radiation burns 128
ramsons 68, **132–5**; harvesting 134; recipes 134
rashes 9, 85, 116, 130, 179, 180
raspberry 11, 17, 18, 102, **136–8**, 196; recipes 138
Raynaud's syndrome 63, 66
recuperation 54, 82, 166, 172, 190
red clover 22, **139–41**; harvesting 141; recipes 141
red poppy xv, 73, **142–5**; recipes 145
reflux 48
relaxation 84, 140, 172, 189, 191
renal colic 124
respiratory tract 36, 71, 112, 117, 145, 174, 177
restless leg 63
retina, detached 10, 11
rheumatism 14, 15, 23, 27, 29, 41, 44, 48, 63, 70, 79, 83, 98, 99, 114, 155, 156, 177, 185, 195
riboflavin 90
Romans 36, 81, 101, 111, 116, 170, 171, 177, 188
*Rosa* spp. **178–83**
rosebay willowherb **146–9**; recipes 149

rosemary 55
rosewater 60, 180
rowan 16
*Rubus fruticosus* **16–19**
*Rumex crispus* **46–9**

S
sacred plant 14, 64, 70, 97, 107, 115, 121, 127, 139, 159, 170, 177
SAD (seasonal affective disorder) 159, 162, 163
sage 72, 111
salad 26, 29, 30, 32, 52, 55, 72, 81, 95, 138, 140, 144, 157, 164
salicylic acid 70, 97, 184–5
*Salix* spp. **184–5**
salvestrols 137
*Sambucus nigra* **56–61**
sanicle 152
saponins 26, 27, 28, 29, 76
saw palmetto 116
scars 39, 41, 162
sciatica 99, 162
Scotland 6, 16, 105, 129, 147
scrofula 140, 151, 171
sedative 73, 84, 140, 144, 145, 176
sekanjabin 103
selenium 90
self-heal xvii, **150–4**, 172, 180, 190; recipes 153–4
shepherd's purse **155–7**; recipes 157
shingles 29, 130, 161, 162
shins 128
shock 149
silica 81, 82
sinuses 79, 191
sinusitis 102
skin: conditions 14, 20, 22, 26–9, 32, 33, 48, 49, 52, 54, 55, 59, 60, 83, 85, 117, 124, 132, 134, 140, 141, 167, 180, 182; creams xvii–xviii, 18
skullcap 71, 73
sleep 144, 160, 177, 189, 191
slimming 28
slippery elm xviii, 27, 99, 128
smoking 36, 107, 140
smoothies 32
smudge stick 106, 109
soothing 94, 95, 177
sores 37, 73, 122, 130, 153
soup 32, 95, 114, 118
South Africa 47, 104, 161
spasm 98, 102, 140, 177, 180
spearmint 100, 102
spirits 14
spleen 48, 52
splinters 27, 64, 112, 113, 174, 175
sports injuries 41, 185
sprains xviii, 4, 39, 41, 59, 83, 94, 162, 197
St John's day 107, 108, 129, 161
St John's wort x, xv, 39, **158–63**, 180, 189; harvesting 162; recipes 162–3
*Stachys officinalis* **188–91**
*Stellaria media* **26–9**
stinging nettle: *see* nettle
stings 27, 47, 53, 114, 115, 116, 127, 130
stomach 134, 185; acid 48, 52, 97–8, 99, 161; nervous 73, 79, 102, 103; ulcers 94, 129, 130

strawberry 9
stress 4, 84, 86, 108, 109, 170, 189, 190
strewing herbs 97, 101
stroke 66
succus xv, 33, 130
sucrose 13
sunburn 27, 33, 48, 59, 161, 195
sunstroke 90
superfood 88
sweating 58, 59, 60, 79, 84, 102, 122, 145, 171–2, 193, 194
Sweet Annie 108
sweet cicely **164–6**; recipes 166
sweets xvii, 144
swellings 94, 95, 112, 153, 155
*Symphytum officinale* **38–41**
syphilis 22
syrups xvi, 8, 11, 15, 18, 24, 25, 58, 69, 79, 81, 83, 96, 124, 125, 148, 149, 170, 180, 183

T
tannins 4, 9, 18, 121, 122, 180
*Taraxacum officinale* **50–5**
Teasel **167–9**; recipes 169
teeth 18, 82, 85, 122, 123, 128
tendonitis 39, 41
tension 5, 84, 85, 86, 108, 172, 189, 191, 193, 196
testosterone 90
thiamine 82
thread veins 77, 88, 91, 196
throat: cancer 93; problems 112, 112, 122, 150, 151, 152; sore 4, 5, 18, 19, 24, 25, 28, 37, 60, 71, 95, 138, 145, 148, 149, 153, 179, 182, 183
thrombosis 66, 68, 193
thyroid 32, 152, 153, 171, 172
tinctures xiv–xv, 5, 10, 11, 20, 25, 33, 49, 54, 59, 63, 69, 73, 77, 86, 91, 108, 109, 118, 119, 130, 141, 144, 145, 156, 157, 162, 169, 170, 172, 177, 185, 191, 196
toffee 23
tonic 15, 18, 30, 32, 33, 69, 73, 81, 90, 102, 114, 117, 118, 132, 134, 167, 174, 191
tonsillitis 31, 33, 71, 122
toothache 95, 102, 185
toxicity xii, 36, 40, 57, 74, 76, 82, 88, 107, 141, 156, 161
toxins 16, 141, 172, 194
Traditional Chinese Medicine (TCM) 3, 48, 71, 87–90, 102, 107, 118, 151, 167
travel sickness 102, 103
*Trifolium pratense* **139–41**
tuberculosis 111, 151, 152
tumors 88, 159
Turner, William 96
*Tussilago farfara* **34–7**
tutsan 162
typhoid dysentery 148

U
ulcers 9, 22, 73, 04, 97, 98, 99, 122, 123, 129, 130, 134, 148, 149, 153, 161
United States 17, 18, 85, 147, 148, 161, 169
urethritis 32, 43, 45, 98
uric acid 14, 22, 25, 98
urinary system 53, 59, 85, 112, 124–5, 174, 179, 187

urinary tract infection 52, 54, 71, 94, 195
urine: bleeding in 152, 156; burning 33, 125
urogenital tract inflammation 9, 11, 14, 32
urva ursi 156
uterine: pain 124, 137, 148, 177, 181, 195; prolapse 155, 190; tonic 174

V
*Vaccinium myrtillus* **6–11**
vaginal discharge 174, 175, 193; infection 3
varicose veins 9, 10, 27, 39, 52, 76–7, 88, 91, 128, 174, 191, 196
*Verbascum* spp. **110–13**
*Verbena officinalis* **170–2**
vertigo 191
vervain ix, 73, 145, 161, **170–2**, 189; harvesting 172; recipes 172
*Viburnum opulus* **62–3**
vinegars xv, xvi, xviii, 29, 79, 103, 138, 183
viral infections 53, 125, 152, 153, 162, 170, 180, 182
vitamin A 8, 25, 26, 27, 52, 57, 179
vitamin B complex 25, 52, 81, 90, 129, 157
vitamin C 8, 25, 26, 27, 52, 88, 90, 114, 137, 157, 179, 183
vitamin D 52
vitamin K 4, 179
vomiting 70, 100
vulva 135

W
Wales 6, 7, 106, 107, 171
warts 52, 167
waters, aromatic 180
white deadnettle **173–5**; harvesting 175; recipes 175
whooping cough 140, 177
wild lettuce 145, **176–7**; recipes 177
wild rose xv, 152, **178–83**; recipes 182–3
willow 97, 147, **184–5**, 186; recipes 185
willowherb **186–7**; harvesting 187; recipe 187
wine xv, 15, 61, 96, 103, 140, 144, 185, 189
witchcraft 111, 129, 189
wood betony 73, 145, **188–91**; harvesting 151; recipes 191
woodbine **70–1**
worms 108
wormwood 104, 106–7
wound herbs 4, 18, 38, 39, 82, 83, 94, 95, 117, 122, 128, 130, 140, 148, 149, 150, 151, 153, 156, 159, 171, 175, 192, 193, 196
woundwort 188
wrinkles 77

XYZ
yarrow 59, 68, 72, 83, 106, 115, 128, 161, **192–6**; harvesting 196; recipes 196
yellow dock 46–9, 141
ylang ylang 55